Soothing Food

Soothing Food

a new view of cooking for ulcers and difficult stomachs

BEN DUNCAN

With a Foreword by
Dr. Robert Kemp, M.D., F.R.C.P.

FABER AND FABER
3 Queen Square
London

First published in 1972
by Faber and Faber Limited
3 Queen Square London WC1
Printed in Great Britain by
Latimer Trend & Co Ltd Plymouth

ISBN 0 571 09158 x

Contents

Foreword

The story of the rise of duodenal ulcer to become a popular illness is a fascinating one. The history of the condition has been covered in my Rogers Prize Essay (University of London) in 1936 under the title of 'The Natural History of Peptic Ulcer'. Until the early years of this century it was unknown and undiagnosed clinically until Lord Moynihan in his book of 1908 put it on the surgical map. In those early years it was not possible to make a diagnosis except by operation though the symptoms and the cases were becoming more frequent. During the first war the condition was hardly mentioned as a cause of disability. For accurate medical diagnosis we had to await the arrival of more sophisticated X-ray machines and the necessary expertise, both of which were hardly perfected before 1930. Thereafter the condition became the most common condition admitted to the medical wards. With the arrival of World War II all the contesting armies were forced to invalid a steady stream of combatants on these grounds. In 1945 one found on returning to civilian hospital life that there were large numbers of troublesome duodenal ulcer cases made worse by rationing, housing and resettlement difficulties. There were many complications and much drastic surgery. It looked as if the ulcer problem would continue to increase indefinitely.

This did not prove to be so, however, and as the post-war situation settled down, so did the ulcers. The surgeons found that they were not called from their beds so often to operate on the perforations and the physicians found that bleeding from the ulcers was less frequent. By the middle 1950s it was clear that the epidemic was receding and ulcers were being replaced in popularity by other illnesses such as coronary thrombosis. Nobody has been able to explain why the ulcers have become less troublesome, even though still quite frequent. It may be that shorter hours, better wages, better housing have helped the patients to give their complaint better care. There can be no doubt, however, that by the 1970s the condition is much more easily managed, there are many fewer patients in need of medical care in the wards and surgical treatment is much less called for and is itself much less drastic.

To one who is not an ulcer patient this improvement, even if unexplained, would seem to be good news. But to the patient it means that his standing as a patient has been devalued and his place on the front page has been taken by upstart illnesses with a self-induced basis such as lung cancer, heart attacks, obesity, alcoholism and drug problems. Such rapid changes in the fashionability of illness has always been a feature of medical history.

Even when duodenal ulcers were in their heyday I never managed to put my finger convincingly on their cause. It is true that there is a strong family tendency, but this is so of many other illnesses. It is also clear that all patients have the capacity for manufacturing in their stomachs a much greater quantity of acid gastric juice than normal people. Various guesses have been made as to why this should be so without, however, any proof, but what seems to happen is that this highly acid gastric juice is extremely liable to burn a small ulcer in the first part of the duodenum. This in turn becomes a chronic condition which is extremely reluctant to heal. One of its useful peculiarities is, however, that though unhealed it can go for long periods without causing any pain.

Foreword

Bouts of ulcer pain are usually started off by worry and frustration, the wrong food, too much beer, aspirin or other irritant drugs. The art then of managing to own a trouble-free ulcer is that of never at any time doing anything that will annoy it. The type of management needed is set out in my *Family Doctor* booklet, 'Making friends with your ulcer', published by the British Medical Association. I have no intention of repeating here what has been said extensively there.

Mr. Duncan's book deals with one aspect of management, namely housekeeping, menu planning, recipes and cookery suitable for the ulcer patient. He realizes that not only must one pander to the stomach but that the owner of the ulcer must also have the pleasure of eating interesting and palatable food. The days of the dull ulcer diet are long past—restrictive diets were never effective because the patient soon gave them up. Indeed, it is best to abandon completely the concept of diet. It is really not very difficult to find interesting and varied meals which suit ulcers. The author here takes the matter even further. He turns the whole subject into an absorbing and fascinating hobby. He has asked me to go carefully through all his recommendations and has cheerfully made amendments on my suggestions. Naturally he has tested his recipes on his own quite sensitive ulcer and I can only admire the way in which he has set out to put his experience to work for other sufferers. In recommending his efforts to ulcer patients I feel that he has significantly helped the campaign for quieter ulcers.

ROBERT KEMP
LIVERPOOL, 1971

Introduction

I have had an ulcer since I was seventeen. A bachelor, I have cooked for myself. During this time, I have often wished for a cookery book to help me. Finally, encouraged by the much broader outlook on diet of the medical profession in recent years, I decided to write it myself.

I have no medical knowledge, apart from that which any ulcer sufferer is bound to collect. I have no more training in diet or nutrition than anyone else with a reasonable education. But I have had twenty-five years of cooking for an ulcer and of enjoying or regretting what I gave myself to eat. This experience is my qualification for writing this book.

It is not, therefore, a book for those under strict instructions from their doctors. Nor should it be used by those who have not sought medical advice about some stomach condition.

Rather, it is for those with diagnosed duodenal ulcers, whose doctors have given them only general advice about food, and who themselves, or whose wives, may find it difficult to put this into practice.

The limitations upon what ulcer sufferers may eat today are not in the least severe. But they still are extra complications to the tasks of planning, shopping for, and cooking meals.

One way to manage is to cook at every meal a separate bland dish for the ulcer patient. It is a bad way. No one who cooks has the vitality to think out, let alone to prepare, two different but successful menus at every meal. The ulcer sufferer will be given poached eggs or plaice baked in milk until he is sick of them, and he will then go out and eat something more interesting, which will upset him.

Another way to manage is, since ideas of diet for ulcers are now so liberal, to decide that those with ulcers can eat anything. Those acting on this principle will not use this book, and therefore are not my concern. I do not envy them.

I know, with the certainty of knowledge acquired unpleasantly, that the only way for someone with an ulcer to lead a comfortable and equable existence is to eat punctually meals prepared with some consideration for his special needs. I have tried to show, in this book, how it can be achieved.

This attempt might be thought a frightening responsibility for someone without obvious credentials. The thought of the number of inevitably uninformed and inexperienced cooks who must every day provide meals for ulcerated stomachs has encouraged me to go on. I have tried, as conscientiously as I can, to supplement my experience by some understanding of the theory involved. I have learned what I can, from books, from my doctors, and from the large number of others with ulcers whom I know. I act on this knowledge in catering for myself, and in this book I put it forward for others who may be new to the subject.

I do so within the traditional framework of the ulcer diet, but loosened as the new climate of opinion warrants, and as my own experience confirms. There is not now, and there never has been, complete agreement among doctors about what those with ulcers should and should not eat. Theories vary from time to time, and from country to country.

I cannot, therefore, state categorically—and nor can anyone else—that this or that must never be eaten. What I can do is to state clearly the limits within which I work, and which I recommend to others. I divide this outline into two parts. The first lists the kinds of food which in my opinion the ulcer sufferer should always avoid. The second draws attention to a more questionable group, about which there is much disagreement. Here, where I have views, I state them.

Foods to be Avoided

All fried foods of any kind, including chips and potato crisps.

All curries, and dishes similarly seasoned with cayenne or other hot spices.

Any cut of meat which is predominantly fat, bone or gristle; any tough meat.

All pickles, relishes, chutneys, or anything else either preserved in vinegar, or containing it.

Most shellfish, particularly mussels, lobster, and crab.

All raw vegetables, unless otherwise stated.

Green or red peppers, whether cooked or raw.

Tinned tomatoes, and most particularly tinned tomato paste.

Unripe or acid fruits.

Commercial meat extracts.

Commercially-prepared meat products such as sausages, meat pies, and pasties.

Baked beans, especially tinned baked beans.

Glazed fruits; nuts; particularly the dried coconut used in the confectionary trade; mincemeat.

Suet or other heavy puddings.

Questionable Foods

Leaf vegetables; tough vegetables; undercooked vegetables.

Pork and its products; game.

Pastry.

Freshly-baked and hot breads.

This short outline is compiled from many lists, consulted over many years, and constantly revised in the light of experience and further reading.

Some lists ban all tomatoes. I find them innocuous and I use them in my recipes. The tinned ones, and above all, the tinned paste, are deadly.

Other lists ban meat stocks. I believe that some confusion exists here. The commercial meat extracts do certainly set off trouble; and a clear broth is not a good soup to set before someone with an ulcer. But a freshly-made light meat or chicken stock, as the basis of a thick soup, a vegetable purée, or a sauce, is in my view a most soothing contribution to the diet.

No one can be dogmatic about leaf vegetables. Sorrel, cabbage, and sprouts I do not eat nor include in this book. Most ulcer patients find that lettuce is safe to eat. I am one of the few who does not, so no recipes for it are included. But no directions are really necessary, except to suggest that the tough outer leaves are best avoided.

For my strict warning against the use of vinegar I have scientific backing. I have none for including my own suggested small quantities of lemon juice, nor for recommending in some recipes that it should be boiled before use. Lemon juice is, and however treated remains, acid. I find it harmless when used precisely as I specify, and in this I am supported by other writers on ulcer diet. But it is not to be used indiscriminately.

I would think the space wasted if I set out what an ulcer sufferer can eat, since this is what the entire book describes. But any cook will see at once that the modern approach to ulcer diet includes almost the whole of the range of foods perhaps most appealing to present-day tastes: eggs, cheese, fish, chicken, lamb and occasionally beef. Few pleasures are denied in vegetables, and a kitchen that does not have the smell of the *Brassica* tribe boiled into its walls is a pleasure in itself.

This list makes clear, too, that there is no conflict whatever between food that will not upset an ulcer, and the providing of family meals. Just occasionally, of course, you may want to give the ulcer sufferer something different. But I have tried to organize the book in such a way that even in difficult periods one main dish will work for everyone.

The first section of the book consists of soups; the second of dishes of a generally bland kind, which can be main courses when the ulcer patient is feeling tender, or can be used as first courses at a party meal, or simply when the main course for some reason is not quite enough. The third section consists of fish dishes, which are also excellent for difficult times. The fourth and longest section contains the main courses which will do for ordinary times.

I then have a short section of Borderline Dishes, to be served when the ulcer has been quiet for a long time and you are looking for some exciting new tastes. These dishes would not have appeared in the old books on ulcer food. You can, if you want to be cautious, avoid them.

But both they, and the organization of recipes I have chosen, seem to me to fit more realistically the genuine case of someone with an ulcer, in a family, with a busy wife looking after him.

To read, as I have done in preparing this book, many works old and new on ulcer diet, and to compare these with the actual eating and drinking habits of those with ulcers I know, brings home the alarming gap between theory and practice.

On the printed page, ulcerated people touch no alcohol, no meat beyond a steamed breast of chicken, no fruit or vegetable not pressed through a hair sieve. I see people with ulcers accepting the third double whiskey. I meet them strolling along, avoiding my eye, and hiding a newspaper parcel which gives off the strong smell of fried fish and vinegar.

My hope, in this book, is to narrow that gap. I am afraid that every ulcer sufferer will go on the occasional foolish spree. But these harmful outings can be kept to a minimum by the provision of carefully-prepared food as interesting as the stomach, at that moment, can take. This, it seems to me, is all a cook can do, and all a book on ulcer cookery can hope to help with.

A home is not a hospital diet kitchen, and too much medical detail proves simply worrying to someone preparing a meal. Some books on the subject grade each recipe according to the degree of healing of the ulcer. I should not find this helpful myself, and to follow that method in this book would lend a spurious air of medical authority quite at odds with the basis of practical experience, which is all I claim for it.

My method does demand of the cook some exercise of judgement. I do not think anyone living under the same roof with an ulcer can fail to know when it is acting up, and when behaving well. Anyone who is in doubt can always ask.

Occasionally, forethought can help. Before a journey, or what is known to be a difficult day ahead at work, a choice from the section of particularly safe dishes would be sensible. Changes of season, or of weather, are times for caution, too.

As well as those sections mentioned already, the book contains a long section of vegetable dishes, a short one on cold food and salads, and a group of sweet dishes.

It does not contain breakfast dishes as such, nor breakfast menus. Looking critically at such sections in other books, and discussing the subject with others who have ulcers, I conclude that people's tastes and habits in the early morning are too varied for me to be able to advise. Instead, I offer at the end of the book a short note on the subject, along with one on the topic of what to drink.

Throughout the book, I have departed from the usual

convention in cookery writing by giving a number of recipes in quantities for two people only. I have always found recipes easier to increase than to divide (what is half of three eggs?).

Meal Times

Meals must be served on time. This point cannot be too much emphasized. Experts may disagree in points of detail about what someone with an ulcer should eat, but all recognize that a missed meal, or even a late meal, can be a disaster. A biscuit, or a piece of bread and butter, is a useful temporary expedient. But do not come to rely on it. The stomach that has been too long fobbed off with these titbits will sometimes decide it must make do with them, and refuse the meal when it comes. A reckoning invariably follows. Please see my note on p. 169.

Whether you eat with your children or not, the meal should be a well-organized and calm occasion, not a cafeteria-style rough-house. I am told by some of my friends with families that this bachelor ideal is impossible to achieve. I visit other houses, often those with no help and not a great deal of money to spare, where parents and children sit down together, on time, in peace, at every meal. The difference is of method, not size of family. The second way is the one to keep an ulcer under control.

Do not delay the meal by a drinking bout. The person with the ulcer cannot, or should not, join in it. If you have guests, they may be surprised nowadays to be given a glass of sherry and told they are going to eat in ten minutes. But they come back, I find. The entertainment is no less pleasant. It is cheaper. The conversation is better, and the ulcer is not made worse.

Cost

A household including someone with an ulcer must spend a

larger part of its income on food than is usual in England. There is no avoiding this fact, and to resist it is to invite trouble. In such a family, whose affairs are well-conducted, a great deal will be saved on smoking and drinking, which helps.

I have tried to help too by introducing as many inexpensive dishes as I can, including some slow-cooking methods for inexpensive cuts of meat which used to be regarded as unsuitable because of their toughness. These all, however, employ lean flesh. The worst of all dishes for the ulcer diet is one that involves a lot of effort for the person eating it, with little solid result: breast cuts of meat, or fish which are all skin and bones. They excite the stomach's expectation for food, and then fail to satisfy it. They are false economies. Far better ones are dishes using rice or pasta to make the expensive protein go further; the cheaper fish; or egg dishes.

Fats

I have specified butter in many recipes. To me, the taste of it makes appealing many otherwise uninteresting ways of cooking. The very cheapest butters, wherever they come from and however blended, work in this way for me, but margarine does not. I cannot therefore recommend it as a substitute. But if you like, or don't mind the taste, then you are not merely allowed by medical opinion to use margarine, you will have the blessing of many doctors concerned about the over-use of dairy fats in diet generally.

Those who prefer butter will find that the quantities I suggest are not excessive, and are perfectly acceptable medically. Those whose doctors give specific advice on this point will obviously follow it.

Of the various cooking and salad oils available, I know no medical opinion that favours one over the others, so you can make your choice on grounds of taste and cost. Olive oil is now very expensive, oils of groundnuts, corn, and sunflower seeds much less so. I keep some olive oil for use when its taste will tell, and sunflower oil for more general use.

Since I do not suggest frying at all in this book, the behaviour of oils when very hot should not arise. But for the light browning of ingredients which I do recommend for long-cooked dishes, or for other cooking of this kind, many reputable cookery writers commend the use of oil and butter mixed. Since this blend is designed to prevent the overheating of the butter, it has dietary as well as culinary advantages.

Finally, although I have implied these rules throughout this book, they are so important that I here state them flatly:

1. The raising to high temperatures (as in deep frying) of oil or other cooking fats must be avoided totally when cooking for those with ulcers.

2. Re-heated cooking fats are particularly dangerous, in the view of many, and in my experience; if you do deep frying, or other such cooking, when the ulcer sufferer is not present, do not re-use these cooking fats on occasions when he is present.

Pre-packed foods

Since so much ulcer cookery is so very time-consuming, the person who does this job should not hesitate to use ingredients in which some of the preparation is already done. These, however, must be chosen with care.

Pre-scrubbed vegetables as sold by good chain stores save much trouble, and cost little more. During the time of year when fresh vegetables are largely limited to sprouts and cabbage, frozen ones can be helpful. Apply to these the same rules—and the same common sense—as to any other vegetables, including the use of the food mill on those with hard skins or hulls. Sweet corn becomes tough when frozen, and is best avoided, on its own or in mixtures.

Doctors give conflicting advice about the safety of frozen meat and fish. A warning is certainly necessary about many commercially frozen products but meat or fish that has been properly deep frozen, thawed and cooked can be perfectly safe. Frozen chicken is not only safe but too useful to be ignored. The instructions for thawing must be followed with particular care by those cooking for the ulcer diet. With this warning, both frozen joints and whole chickens can be used in many recipes in this book, apart from the one or two which specify them. A useful book on all aspects of home freezing is *Deep Freezing* by Pat M. Cox.

Tins are especially welcome in emergencies, but have other uses, too. The dangerous exception, which cannot be stated too often, is any tin containing tomatoes or tomato paste; or even the many prepared tinned foods such as spaghetti, which contain this most upsetting substance.

Certain dried foods, such as lentils, can be useful if put through the food mill. But the commercially-packed quick-dried foods I have tried often contained tough pieces, and in consequence I think the products of this method of preserving unsuitable for use in the ulcer diet.

I would, in general, be on the lookout for any genuinely time-saving advances in pre-packing of food, provided they fall within the scheme of the diet, and that the foods don't lose their own flavours in the process. This last is a point of general importance. If you have an ulcer, and therefore don't go in for heavy smoking, drinking, or harsh seasonings like vinegar and horseradish, you know what food tastes like, and you mind. No food is worth including in this diet which an ulcer sufferer will pick at, or refuse.

Equipment

Almost all ulcer cookery takes time and trouble, and more of these the less the meal costs. Good equipment helps to cut down kitchen time.

An electric blender is undoubtedly a great advantage, but is not worth bankrupting the household to buy. No recipe in this book requires it, though many are made easier by it. If not a blender, then some other good way to mill fruit and vegetables is necessary. The French Moulin-Légumes is the only one I know of that is big enough to take reasonable quantities, efficient, and easy to wash. It is called the Mouli by most people who use it, and by me in this book. It is much to be recommended.

Otherwise, all of what is needed should be in any well-run kitchen: knives that can really be sharpened, a chopping-board, soufflé dishes, and at least one dish that can be used on direct heat as well as in the oven. Good kitchen shops now sell many versions. They also sell other time-saving gadgets and pieces of equipment, some of which I suggest in connection with certain recipes.

Some cooks find pressure cookers invaluable; others, uncongenial. I'm the second kind, so I do not include recipes in this book. But I can reassure those who like pressure cookers that doctors commend them for ulcer cookery.

Seasoning

Seasoning by infusion is an important process in ulcer cookery. Pepper, or other ground spices, or even dried herbs, must be used sparingly, for the pieces themselves can upset. But whole spices, or herbs, put into a dish to season it, and removed before serving, are harmless. Where they would not be sieved out anyway, it is convenient either to use a small tea infuser, or to tie the herbs or spices in a small piece of the cheesecloth which most department stores sell.

Of the spices and seasonings themselves, the important ones are: (1) black peppercorns, not white ones which are hotter and less aromatic; (2) bay leaves; (3) whole allspice, whole cloves, whole nutmeg, mace, stick cinnamon and juniper berries.

Flavouring herbs assume some importance in a kitchen where hot peppery bottled sauces and vinegar-based preserves play no part. They help to make simple food more varied and appealing, and add interest for the cook, too.

Good dried herbs are now sold in this country, and work satisfactorily in long-cooked dishes. Fresh herbs are not so easy to buy, but they are not much trouble to grow if you have a little piece of ground, or even the space for pots or window boxes.

If I were short of space, I should limit myself to these three, for their usefulness in cooking for someone with an ulcer:

1. A good supply of the flat-leaved Hamburg parsley, *Petroselinum sativum*, also called French or Italian parsley. Much easier to wash than curly parsley, it also tastes more strongly, so less can be used.

2. A good plant of the true French tarragon, bought from a reliable plant nursery.

3. Thyme of some kind.

Basil and chervil are exquisite, both can be grown in pots, but are short-lived and temperamental. Dill or fennel is worth having, but takes up a lot of room. Fresh sage is nicer than the dried form suggests. It, and rosemary, grow as shrubs in many gardens; if you don't have them, consider them, or see if your neighbour has them and will spare the occasional branch.

Sources

A book of this kind poses particular problems of attribution. Although many recipes are completely my own, many more have been taken from other cookery books and altered to a greater or lesser extent to suit them to this book's special requirements. I have no wish to claim some other writer's work as my own. Yet I cannot either attribute to someone else a recipe I have changed.

In the few cases where I have found a recipe I can use

outright, I have noted its source. Otherwise I can only make general acknowledgements, which I do in the Bibliography at the end. This includes notes of those books that seem to me worth either having, or consulting, in a household where there is an ulcer.

I am especially grateful to Isabella Menzies and Fortune Stanley, who most generously allowed me to see before publication their collection *A Book of Edwardian Food*, and to use recipes from it. A number of public bodies were helpful, particularly the White Fish Authority, and the Herring Industry Board. The librarian of India House was of real assistance to me in the section on rice. My neighbour, Clare Chapman, gave me encouragement and practical help throughout.

Finally, my connection with Scurfield, the pioneer kitchen shop in Cambridge, has been of much use, and many members of its staff, past and present, have supplied me with information and ideas. Its present owner, Dick Chapman, has not only helped me in every possible way, but has also, for the two years I have taken to complete the book, eaten uncomplainingly my successful and less successful attempts at ulcer cookery.

Recipes

Soups

1. Avgolemono soup
2. Carrot vichyssoise
3. Leek and potato soup
4. Vichyssoise
5. Mushroom soup
6. Jerusalem artichoke soup
7. Cauliflower soup
8. Cream of tomato and orange
9. Cream of vegetable soup
10. Borsch

INTRODUCTION

The association of broths with invalid cookery is a misleading one. A clear soup or consommé, or broths with vegetables or pasta floating in them, should not be given to someone with an ulcer, particularly when unwell; nor, at any time, the commercial meat extracts which their manufacturers suggest for convalescents; nor any soup based upon these. (Soups served in public eating places, which may contain them, are therefore always suspect.)

A thick, nourishing soup is best. Such soups, which are filling, should not overwhelm a possibly doubtful appetite. A small quantity is enough, and something should follow which will keep the meal well-balanced, even if small-scale.

Although almost all the soups in the section that follows contain stock, I've given no directions for it, simply because so much cookery for those with ulcers produces flavoursome liquids: boiled beef or chicken, steamed vegetables, many others. These, strained, reduced, with all fat removed, will provide quite enough stock for as many soups as most people will want.

1. Avgolemono Soup

1 *pint stock*	½ *small lemon*
1 *egg*	1 *tablespoon rice*

The name of this soup simply joins together the Greek words for egg and lemon.

The best stock for it by far is the liquid from a boiled chicken. The liquid should be strained, cooled, left in the refrigerator overnight, and have all fat removed from the top.

The making of the soup cannot be done in advance, nor can the finished soup be kept waiting.

Bring stock to the boil and cook the rice in it for 20 minutes. Meanwhile, beat the egg and the lemon juice together with an egg whisk. When the rice is cooked, remove the pan from the fire and add the hot stock to the beaten egg and lemon juice—but add no more than a tablespoon at a time, stirring well. When about half is added, pour the mixture in the bowl slowly into the remaining stock in the pan. Stir thoroughly together, return to the fire and slowly heat up again. Do not allow to boil. When the soup is heated through, it will thicken a little, and should then be served at once.

2. Carrot Vichyssoise

This soup is thick and nourishing, and contains enough vegetables for the whole meal, which should be planned accordingly.

4 *carrots*
2 *potatoes*
2 *leeks*
1 *pint stock*
1 *pint milk*
4 *peppercorns*
salt

Peel and slice the carrots and potatoes. Remove every bit of green leaf from the leeks. Split them, wash them very carefully, cut them into small squares.

Simmer the vegetables in the stock with a little salt and 4 peppercorns. When the vegetables are soft (35–40 minutes) put the whole mixture through the Mouli. If you use a food blender instead, fish out the peppercorns first. Reheat, adding the milk gradually. Do not boil again, and serve when heated through.

3. Leek and Potato Soup

This soup has a reputation I think it deserves for settling and calming ulcers.

Many slightly varying recipes exist for it, as Potage Bonne Femme, Potage Parmentier, or Hot Vichyssoise. I advance my own because (1) some I've tried contain too high a proportion of potatoes, (2) I don't like putting the odd carrot in it, but prefer making the completely separate soup really tasting of carrots, which precedes this one, (3) my version forms the basis of the best cold soup for the ulcer diet, which follows this one.

1½ *lb. leeks after preparation*
  (2–2½ *lb. when bought*)
½ *lb. potatoes*
1½–2 *pints chicken stock*
2 *tablespoons butter*
peppercorns
salt
milk
parsley

The weights above should mean about eight medium-sized leeks to two small potatoes. Remove every bit of green leaf from the leeks. Split and wash them very carefully. Peel and slice the potatoes.

Warm the leeks over a low heat in the butter for 5 minutes, add the potatoes and cook for another 5. Gradually add the stock, 4 peppercorns, a teaspoon of salt, and cook until tender: 35–40 minutes.

Put it into a blender, if you have one, fishing out the peppercorns first. If you use a Mouli, you may have to put the mixture through twice to get out all the lumps.

Before serving, reheat, add the top off a bottle of milk, and a handful of finely chopped parsley.

4. Vichyssoise (Crème Vichyssoise Glacée)

ingredients from preceding recipe (except milk and parsley)
8 oz. cream
chives

To make my simplified form of this delicious Franco-American soup, you use precisely the previous one, but instead of heating it up with milk and parsley, you cool it and finish it differently.

They taste so unlike that you can, if you want, make enough for two goes, serve the hot soup one day and the cold a day or so after: both suit the time in autumn when leeks first appear and the weather is neither hot nor cold.

So: make the soup as described above, all but the final reheating. Chill in the refrigerator, and just before serving add the cream and stir well. Putting the soup bowls in the refrigerator to chill is worth doing; so is saving a little cream to put a drop in the centre of each bowl. Cut the chives finely over this.

5. Mushroom Soup

½ *lb. mushrooms*
1 *pint milk*
1 *pint water*
3 *tablespoons flour*
4 *tablespoons butter*
bacon rinds or 1 *bacon rasher*
6 *peppercorns*
salt

Many mushroom soup recipes suit the ulcer diet, but this one produces more well-flavoured soup from fewer mushrooms than most.

Make a white sauce with the butter, flour and milk. While this cooks, bring 1 pint of water to the boil and put in the well-washed mushrooms, whole, the bacon rinds or rasher, 6 peppercorns, and salt.

Cook them for 7 minutes. Strain the mushrooms, keeping

the water, and add this gradually to the white sauce, stirring well. Remove the bacon and peppercorns from the mushrooms. Chop the mushrooms fairly finely, or put them with a little of the sauce into a blender for only a few seconds. Add to the sauce. When ready to serve, heat through, taste, and add salt if necessary.

6. Jerusalem Artichoke Soup

1–1½ lb. Jerusalem artichokes
1 pint mild stock
⅓ pint cream or *top of milk*
salt

Stock from chicken or other poultry is best.

Scrub the artichokes well with a brush. Boil them for 10 minutes in water, then peel with a table-knife when they are cool enough to handle. Put them into the stock and simmer for 20 minutes. Put the whole mixture through the Mouli, or into a blender. When ready to serve, re-heat, bring the cream or top of milk to the boil, and add to the mixture. Taste, and add salt, before serving.

The blender, and cream, produce a professional-looking result; the Mouli, and milk, a more home-made appearance.

7. Cauliflower Soup

1 medium-sized cauliflower
1½ pints stock
¼ pint milk
2 oz. butter
4 egg yolks
salt

Remove the leaves of the cauliflower and separate it into sprigs. Boil it in ¼ inch of water with ¼ teaspoon of salt for 10–15 minutes. Put it through the Mouli, add to the stock, bring to the boil and simmer for 15 minutes. Take off the burner, add the milk, then the butter, stirring well. Whisk the yolks with 4 tablespoons water and add to the soup gradually, stirring as you do. Return the soup to the lowest heat, and stir as it thickens. Don't let it boil, or it will curdle. Taste for salt, but add no pepper, and serve.

Since cauliflowers vary greatly in size, you must obviously alter the quantities if you use either a very small, or an enormous one.

8. Cream of Tomato and Orange

1½ *pints chicken* or *other light stock*
1 *lb. tomatoes*
1 *orange*
1 *carrot*
1 *onion*
4 *tablespoons cream* or *top of milk*
3 *tablespoons butter*
3 *tablespoons flour*
a cube of sugar
seasonings

Wash the tomatoes, remove their stems, halve them and put them into the stock with the peeled and sliced carrot and onion, a bay leaf, 6 peppercorns, and ½ a teaspoon of salt. Wash and dry an orange, take off a very thin strip of peel a couple of inches long, and add this to the stock and vegetables. Keep the orange for later. Simmer the vegetables in the stock for about ¾ hour, then put the whole mixture through the Mouli (a blender will not do). While the mixture is still hot, quickly rinse and dry the pan, and in it melt the butter, add the flour, and blend over a low heat for 3 minutes.

Gradually add the soup mixture off the burner. Return to the burner and cook gently for 10 minutes while stirring. If preparing the soup for later, stop at this point.

Near the time of serving, heat the soup gently, and meanwhile rub a cube of sugar over the orange until all facets are a dark orange colour from the oil. Add the cube to the soup, and when it has dissolved, gradually add the cream or top of milk. Taste, add salt if necessary, and serve.

9. Cream of Vegetable Soup

1 pint stock, water or *milk*
onion
carrots
potatoes
other vegetables as available, to weigh 1 lb. in all
seasonings

To insist upon too precise a recipe would offend against good household management, because the use of this soup is to turn to good account one of the light meat or chicken stocks which so many recipes in this book produce; or the water from steamed vegetables; or the leftover vegetables themselves.

The vegetables, in the proportion of 1 lb. to 1 pint of liquid, should be simmered in it until tender; or if already cooked, just heated through. They should then be put through the Mouli or into a blender. If the consistency produced is not pleasing, either thin the soup by the addition of heated milk, or thicken it. You can do this by any method you feel at home with; I know no way of thickening soups which is harmful to ulcers. Some of the methods I use are described in earlier recipes in this section, but usually, in practice, since so many root vegetables thicken liquids themselves, nothing additional is needed.

Recipes which come with blenders suggest quick ways of making these soups, such as mixing the cooked vegetables with milk in the blender. These methods are safe for this diet, provided they employ the right vegetables.

Seasonings in these thick soups always need a last-minute check. A scattering of finely chopped parsley or other herb improves them, as does a tablespoon of butter, or of cream, stirred in at the last minute.

The most carefully-made vegetable soup occasionally ends up tasting of almost nothing. A very little grated nutmeg sometimes revives it; or one small tomato, washed, cut up, put raw through the Mouli, and then well stirred in.

Good vegetables for thick vegetable soups:

- 1 onion, but not more for the quantity of soup suggested
- carrots
- celeriac
- celery
- Jerusalem artichokes
- leeks, white parts only
- potatoes
- young turnips

Green leaf vegetables, not to be used for soup (or anything else in the ulcer diet):

- cabbage
- sorrel
- spinach
- sprouts
- watercress

Cauliflower doesn't blend well with other vegetable flavours, but is best used on its own for soup (p. 32); so are mushrooms (p. 31), which turn vegetable creams a muddy colour.

10. Borsch

1 *lb. cooked beetroot*
¾–1 *pint strong beef stock* or
1 *tin good beef consommé*
yoghourt or *sour cream*
salt

This version, which uses the cooked beetroot available everywhere, is better for the ulcer diet than the more usual beetroot broth made with the raw vegetable.

The liquid from a boiled beef (p. 103) is ideal; one of the good tinned consommés works extremely well. Chicken stock, or any other not strongly flavoured, is no use.

Peel the cooked beetroot (bought from a trustworthy greengrocer), and remove any imperfections. Dice it roughly.

Heat it up in the stock, put it through the Mouli or into the blender. Salt well, tasting as you do.

When ready to serve, heat the soup through thoroughly. Pour into heated bowls, with a couple of teaspoons of sour cream or yoghourt in the centre of each; or serve this separately.

First Courses and Main Dishes in Time of Trouble

11. Boiled eggs
12. Coddled eggs
13. Scrambled eggs
14. Poached eggs
15. Eggs in ramekins
16. Kitchener eggs
17. Baked omelet
18. Baked egg dishes
19. Eggs in buns
20. Steamed soufflés
21. Steamed ham soufflé
22. Steamed cheese soufflé
23. Steamed rabbit soufflé
24. Pasta in butter
25. Pasticcio
26. A simple risotto
27. Kedgeree
28. Haddock soufflé
29. Cauliflower cheese
30. Stuffed courgettes

INTRODUCTION

The recipes here are arranged more or less in order of mildness, starting with those for times when the ulcer is upset, or is likely to be. Inevitably, these will be the least interesting to other people, and I cannot claim that families or friends will be excited to be given a first course of boiled eggs. But most dishes in this section are of the kind that can be used to begin a substantial meal, or to be the mainstay of a lighter one.

The notion of a 'light' meal for someone with an ulcer can be overdone. A stomach in difficulty can be upset as much by being given too little to work on, as by being given more than it can handle. Unless you have good reason not to, I believe in continuing to offer, even if only a little is accepted of each, the elements of a balanced meal: something from this section, some vegetable, some appropriately simple sweet dish.

Since this is the section to be turned to in times of trouble, it is the place to say again that a stomach which is in serious difficulty is the concern of a doctor, not a cookery writer. If you have anything more than routine difficulties to deal with, don't rely upon recipes, but seek medical advice.

Eggs

This book is not intended for use during an acute attack, when your doctor's advice must be sought. But you will have lesser crises to deal with, and for them simply-cooked eggs will be your best recourse.

I have given some ways I rely on, starting with the safest and moving on to some for better times (pp. 46–49). Since egg cookery may suddenly assume great importance, I believe in having plenty of equipment: a saucepan small enough to boil eggs in without their rattling about, a piercer to make them less likely to crack, even a gadget for slicing the top off neatly. Fussy though this sounds, it may make a difference between an attractively presented egg which will be eaten, and a messy one which won't. Poachers, ramekins, and other gadgets are also suggested in the recipes.

Pasta

The simple forms of pasta—macaroni, noodles, spaghetti, tagliatelle—are excellent foods for delicate stomachs. The kinds stuffed with meat, such as ravioli and cannelloni, should be avoided. Their makers often include tough bits of meat, skin, gristle, even bone; and put them up in strongly-flavoured greasy sauces.

You may be lucky enough to live where you can buy freshly-made pasta containing eggs. Or you may be skilful enough to make your own. Such pasta is so good it needs only the simplest of cooking, such as I suggest in the recipe on p. 50. In any case, no way of cooking pasta is permitted which includes anchovies or other trimmings which are themselves upsetting; cheese baked into an impenetrable crust; or sauces which are virtually fry-ups. Tinned tomato paste will cause instant and prolonged upset; do not use it.

Many cookery books include good recipes which avoid these dangers. I include here only two. The first, for pasta in butter (p. 50), is the dish to serve to a really ailing stomach. The second recipe, the Greek dish Pasticcio (p. 51), forms the basis of a good family meal.

Rice

In every ulcer sufferer's life there are frequent, not medically serious, but troublesome periods when he is wary of eating almost anything for fear of its consequences.

Few of us at such a time will refuse a dish of plain boiled rice, and nothing could be safer. A little butter, a sprinkling of some mild grated cheese, a poached egg on top of the rice can represent a real step towards recovery.

Even in happier times, rice is, I think, the most valuable single food for dealing with an ulcer. I don't think I pass a single week of my life without eating it, and I always have a selection of these in the house:

1. Indian rice, of which the kind I have settled on is one called *basmatti* (the spelling varies). It cooks quickly—in 10–12 minutes from the time it is dropped into rapidly boiling water. It also overcooks quickly. It has a taste of its own, which makes it the obvious choice when nothing is to be used to flavour it. Kedgeree is best made with it.

It often contains grit, if not small pebbles, so it must be picked over carefully before cooking. After cooking, a quick wash in a sieve in very hot water, and a period drying in a low oven improve *basmatti* rice.

2. Italian rice, which cooks slowly and is therefore less likely to come to harm when you can't give it your undivided attention. It absorbs tastes well, and so is the basis of risotto and other dishes in which the rice is cooked in stock, and forms the background for other ingredients. It also makes the best rice salads.

I have for fifteen years used an almost foolproof variety called *avorio*, which I cook slowly for 20–25 minutes, tasting to see when it is tender, and rinsing in hot water in a sieve.

3. Carolina rice, which is often marketed in this country in a prepared form especially easy to cook, and is therefore a worthwhile standby in the kitchen.

4. The rices from various places of origin which are intended to fall apart in nursery puddings, which do so and are therefore essential to these dishes.

I deliberately avoid controversy, since it is bad for ulcers. So I deliberately avoid any directions for cooking rice more specific than those given above. The best method is the one that suits your temperament, and which you can therefore follow successfully. No rigid rules can be laid down. To anyone who thinks they can, I recommend the intelligent summary of conflicting opinions in *Rice Cooking*, by Robin Howe.

Rabbit

Rabbit, as the cheapest of the light, tender meats, featured importantly in the older works on ulcers, and still turns up on hospital diet sheets. However, after the reduction in number by myxamatosis and the rise of the chicken-breeding industry, someone cooking for an ulcer and a family may look more sceptically at the claims of the rabbit.

The best, fresh (not frozen) domestic rabbits can cost more per pound than frozen joints of boiling chicken. A rabbit involves waste: the back legs provide two good helpings, the back, or saddle can be divided into another two, but the forequarters have almost no meat on them.

More important is the unspoken truth that many people are sickened by the taste of rabbit. Recipes for the old invalid diets involved soaking the rabbit for hours in salted water, and then presenting it in some white sauce, as a blanquette or a fricassée. These always seemed to me to emphasize the curious taste that some people dislike, and no attempt to disguise rabbit as chicken actually works.

Therefore, if the ulcer sufferer or anyone else in your family doesn't like rabbit, my advice is not to serve it.

However, some people, and families whom I know positively like rabbit; and there may well still be some areas where it is cheaper than chicken.

I therefore give two representative recipes. One, in this section (p. 49), is a pleasant dish of the old bland school, for periods when the stomach is troublesome. The other, a more robust dish for better times, is on p. 91.

Soufflés

Nothing pleases a troubled ulcer so much as a soufflé. So, if you make them easily you can serve them sure that they will do nothing but good.

If you find them alarming, try the haddock soufflé on p. 54. It is, I think, the easiest of all to make: not the fluffiest, but much more stable than most. (I find that the hardest part of soufflé-making is getting people to the table to eat it.)

As first courses, and for difficult periods, the range of soufflés is almost limitless. The base, to which the beaten whites are added, can be flavoured with cheese, of course. It can be blended with the purées of many vegetables such as young marrows. Sweet soufflés are also useful for adding substance to an otherwise thin meal.

11. Boiled Eggs

For an upset ulcer sufferer, an egg is better boiled lightly, for not more than 3 minutes. But it is no use at all if the patient won't eat it, so cook it for the length of time you know will produce an egg that will be received well; preferably not more than 4 minutes.

Don't, of course, put an egg straight from the refrigerator into fast-boiling water. Don't in any case let the water boil hard, but just simmer, to cook the egg evenly. Don't serve pepper with it, just salt and pieces of thinly-sliced white bread with the crusts removed, toasted, and allowed to cool before they are buttered.

Although it seems too obvious to say, two boiled eggs are better than one for a person who is going to eat nothing else, so a pair is always worth suggesting.

12. Coddled Eggs

These are simply put into water which has just boiled and been taken off the heat. They are supposed to be even more delicate and digestible than boiled eggs. Perhaps they are. I'm not sure that the difference exists.

But coddling is of use if your cooker, like many, has no heat between a cold burner and an inferno. Experts say that four minutes of coddling equals three of boiling. Six minutes will coddle an egg to my taste.

13. Scrambled Eggs

To cook scrambled eggs over boiling water, in a double saucepan or in something you contrive yourself, is safer for the ulcer diet and better cooking practice than to put a pan on direct heat. Precisely how much butter you add, and whether you include either cream or top of the milk, should be decided according to what your household prefers.

14. Poached Eggs

Eggs for poaching mustn't be stale, or the whites fall apart. I use a frying-pan of water, just below boiling, and poaching-rings to keep the eggs in shape. If you can produce a better-looking result by the more sophisticated method of making a whirlpool with a spoon and sliding the egg into it, by all means do so. Don't, however, acidulate the water with vinegar when poaching eggs for an ulcer sufferer, and leave the salting to be done by him. About 5 minutes is the usual time for cooking, or until you can see that the white has set.

Drain each egg well in a slotted spoon, and rest this for a moment on a paper towel to absorb some of the water.

Serve it on buttered toast if you know this way is a

favourite. I much prefer, when my own stomach is troublesome, to eat one or two poached eggs on top of some well-cooked buttered rice.

I suggest also:

1. Poached eggs on a bed of any of the vegetable purées, pp. 119–123; or, when times are a little better, on some non-puréed vegetable, such as steamed carrots.

Do *not* serve, and if you are an ulcer sufferer do not order in a restaurant, Oeufs Florentine, which are poached eggs served on a bed of spinach, and in my view upsetting.

2. Poached eggs served either on puréed or other vegetables are improved by a small quantity of well-seasoned white sauce.

3. Poached eggs can be put into a warmed dish, have poured over them a cheese sauce (p. 160), and be served with toast or bread. Directions for this recipe, called Oeufs Mornay, sometimes say to brown the dish under a grill. For the ulcer diet this direction, which produces a crust and overcooks the eggs, should not be followed.

15. Eggs in Ramekins

The little fireproof dishes that hold one egg provide another useful variation. They can be used in the oven, but the timing is so perilous—and can so easily result in either a late meal or rock-hard eggs which no ulcer sufferer should eat—that I don't recommend it.

A better way is to put the ramekins into any wide pan with a lid, in which the water, only just boiling, comes half way up them. Put a little butter into each ramekin, and when it melts, the egg. Put the lid on the pan, and look after three minutes to see if the whites are set. If they are, the eggs are ready to serve. A tablespoon of double cream added a moment after the egg, turns this into a most delicious and settling dish for the ulcer, or any other, diet.

16. Kitchener Eggs

Good kitchen shops sell little earthenware containers with screw lids called Kitchener egg cups. I believe, despite the spelling difference, that these are linked with the remarkable William Kitchiner, M.D., who from the 1820s onwards published *Peptic Precepts*, and *The Cook's Oracle*, as well as works upon the human eye, vocal music and locomotion. However, I cannot trace the connection. Be that as it may, Kitchener egg cups, far from being mere curiosities, cook eggs excellently. You put into them butter, the egg, and salt (no pepper for the ulcer sufferer). You screw on the lid, put them into a pan of slowly boiling water for 5 minutes, and serve them just as they are, in the cups.

A very little cream can be added, and a small quantity of some delicate herb—chervil, tarragon or basil—will reveal its flavour in this as in no other way. Parsley, mixed with a very few finely chopped chives, makes a pleasant seasoning. Guests, I find, enjoy discovering Kitchener eggs, mothers tell me children like them, and for conveying an egg still hot on an invalid tray I've found nothing to equal them.

A similar egg cup exists in heat-proof clear glass, which to my eye is much less appealing, but it works satisfactorily.

17. Baked Omelet

4 *eggs*
½ *teaspoon salt*
3 *tablespoons hot water*
2 *teaspoons butter*

'Separate eggs. Beat yolks with salt and hot water until thick and pale. Beat egg whites until stiff, and fold them into the yolk mixture. Butter a heavy frying pan and heat in the oven to the foamy stage. Turn in eggs, spreading evenly. Place pan in moderate oven (350°), and cook until omelet is just firm when pressed with the finger. With the aid of a spatula disengage from sides and bottom of pan and slide on to a warm serving-dish without folding. Serves 4.'

I quote the recipe for this excellent way of treating eggs exactly as it appears in *Good Food for Bad Stomachs*, a useful volume described on p. 173. Many English kitchens now have pans, of cast iron, steel, or earthenware, which for this recipe would work better than a frying pan, and can themselves be brought to the table. The dish takes, in my oven, 10–15 minutes, and two people finish it easily.

18. Baked Egg Dishes

These dishes are cheap and easy and useful for times when you have to prepare a meal in a hurry using what happens to be in the larder. The exact timing and oven temperature must be adjusted to your own cooker. I give first a typical recipe, and then list some variations:

4 *eggs*
4 *small tomatoes*
½ *lb. Cheddar* or *other mild English cheese*
1 *cup milk*
butter
salt

Dip the tomatoes in boiling water and peel them. Cut them in half and remove the hard fibrous stem. Chop them, and grate the cheese.

Butter a shallow ovenproof dish. Spread the chopped tomatoes in it and the grated cheese. Break the eggs carefully into the dish and pour over the milk. Add salt.

Put uncovered into a pre-heated oven set at 400°. After the first 15 minutes peep at the dish: the eggs should be set but the yolks should not be hard. This will take 25 minutes, more or less.

The eggs, cheese and milk are the essentials of the dish. Other ingredients can vary according to the season and what you happen to have. Here are some suggestions:

1. ¼ lb. mushrooms, washed and with their stems removed.

2. ½ a small head of very young celery, scrubbed, blanched in boiling water for 5 minutes and cut into inch lengths.

3. Either mushrooms or celery, in half the quantity stated, with two tomatoes.

4. Leftovers of cooked vegetables: leeks, carrots, peas. If these are in large pieces, either chop them on a board or put them through the Mouli. If they provide too bumpy a surface, the yolks will break when you put in the eggs.

19. Eggs in Buns

rolls
grated cheese
eggs
butter
a sauce, see below

Slice the top off a fresh dinner roll, about a third of the way down, and with a teaspoon scoop out as much of the inside as will come away leaving a solid shell. Into the roll put ½ a teaspoon of butter and a teaspoon of any mild grated cheese. Put the rolls like this into the oven pre-heated to 400°, for only 2 minutes, so that they harden, and the cheese and butter melt.

Divide yolks from whites, putting whites together in a bowl, and one yolk into the hole in each roll, with a little salt and pepper. Whisk the whites well, and then quickly fold through them a level tablespoon of cheese to each white. Also quickly, fill the rolls with the whipped whites, and pile up the rest on top of each. Sprinkle a little salt on each. Put at once into the still-hot oven. In 7–10 minutes the whites should be firm and just browning, and the eggs are ready to serve.

A sauce is a great improvement: simply ½ pint of white sauce (p. 160) for every 2–3 eggs, into which you Mouli 2 fresh raw tomatoes, and cook for 5 minutes.

For a first course one bun per person is enough. To make a meal of them you'll obviously want more.

20. Steamed Soufflés

The standard way to steam a soufflé is to prepare a soufflé dish or cake tin by tying around it a double piece of greaseproof paper to project 2 or 3 inches above; and after filling it with the soufflé mixture, to put another square of buttered greaseproof paper on top to stop the steam from watering the soufflé. You set this dish on a steaming rack in a large pan, and keep the water just boiling while the soufflé cooks.

My own method is simply to fit an earthenware bowl or dish of the right size into an extra-large saucepan of water, cover it with a piece of foil and, again, keep the water only barely on the boil.

The first way produces the attractive bursting-over-the-top look when you remove the paper to serve it. My method doesn't, but is less trouble. If you use mine, make due allowance for the rise of the soufflé. For instance, in the recipe that follows a dish of 2½–3 pint capacity is necessary.

Whatever method you use, you must make all preparations in advance, not be trying to tie on bits of paper or fill saucepans while beaten egg whites wait.

A steamed soufflé is, obviously, not so light and exquisite as a proper, quickly-baked one. But it suits the rough-and-tumble of everyday life much better—10 minutes one way or the other doesn't matter, and you can, shocking as it sounds, reheat it the next day, in the oven, sitting it in a pan of water.

21. Steamed Ham Soufflé

½ *lb. ham, minced finely*
1 *pint creamy milk*
2 *tablespoons butter*
2 *tablespoons flour*
¼ *lb. mild Cheddar, grated*
4 *eggs*
seasoning

By creamy milk I mean simply the Channel Island kind bottled with a gold cap.

Remove all fat from the ham and mince it. Grate the cheese. Blend the butter and flour over a low heat, while the milk is heating separately. Add milk slowly to make a smooth white sauce. Let it cool a little, add the ham, the cheese, the egg yolks, and seasonings, and blend well. Keep whites in the refrigerator.

All this can be done in advance. An hour before mealtime, get ready the pan for steaming as described opposite. Fill it with an inch or so of water, bring to the boil and turn down. Beat the egg whites stiff but not dry and fold them into the prepared mixture. Pour into the soufflé dish and steam 40–45 minutes until top feels spongy.

22. Steamed Cheese Soufflé

2 *tablespoons butter*
3 *tablespoons flour*
½ *pint milk*
3 *eggs*
3 *oz. grated mild English cheese*
seasonings

Blend the flour into the butter over a low heat, remove from burner and add gradually the warmed milk. Add the egg yolks, beaten well with 1 tablespoon of water, the grated cheese, salt, a little pepper and some grated nutmeg. Fold in the stiffly-beaten egg whites, and steam the soufflé as described in the preceding recipe.

23. Steamed Rabbit Soufflé

½ *lb. raw lean rabbit, weighed when removed from bone*
1 *oz. butter*
1 *oz. flour*
¼ *pint milk*
seasonings
2 *eggs*
1 *tablespoon cream* or *top of milk*

With a sharp knife cut only lean meat, no membrane or gristle, from the raw rabbit. This is a tedious job, but enables you to make use of the bony front half of the rabbit which poulterers and fishmongers will sometimes sell at a cut price. Two such pieces will be needed to get the right amount of meat. Put the pieces into a bowl of salted water containing a teaspoon of vinegar and leave them an hour or so.

With butter, flour and milk make a white sauce; add salt, a little pepper and a little grated nutmeg. Leave to cool.

Strain the pieces of rabbit, put them through the finest blade of the mincer, and mix them, the yolks of the eggs and the cream or top of milk into the cooled sauce. Whisk the egg whites, fold them lightly in and steam the soufflé as described in a previous recipe. The top should be firm to the touch in ¾–1 hour.

This unexciting but useful dish is more interesting, particularly to those not requiring a bland diet, if served with a separate sauce. Two perfectly acceptable ones for the ulcer sufferer too are a white sauce (p. 160) with one raw tomato, put through the Mouli, added when the sauce has thickened; or one made with a tablespoon or two of finely chopped mushrooms (which can be stems) added to the butter before the flour.

24. Pasta in Butter

¼ lb. pasta per person | *cheese*
butter

Use macaroni, noodles, spaghetti, or tagliatelle.

If you have bought some special quick-cooking kind, follow the cooking instructions on the pack. Otherwise, take ¼ lb. of pasta per person. Have ready a really large pan of boiling water—not less than 1½ quarts per ¼ lb. Do not break the pasta, but feed it gradually into the rapidly boiling water. Turn down the heat, and cook for 15–20 minutes, tasting toward the end to be sure you do not overcook it.

Turn out to drain in a colander, rinsing quickly through with very hot water. Rinse the pan too, and put into it 1 dessertspoon of butter for each serving. Mix butter through pasta with a fork, returning briefly to a low fire, but *do not let the pasta fry*. As soon as the butter is melted serve.

Serve with grated cheese.

25. Pasticcio

1 *lb. macaroni*
1 *lb. minced meat* (*see recipe*)
1 *small onion*
2 *tomatoes*
¼ *cup stock* or *water*
4 *eggs*
4 *oz. grated cheese*
2 *tablespoons olive oil*
butter
cinnamon
nutmeg
sugar
salt
1 *pint Béchamel sauce* (*see p.* 160)

A Greek dish, in effect a macaroni cheese, made more interesting and scarcely more expensive by the layer of meat inside it. This can be beef, lamb or veal, but must contain no bone or gristle.

Put 2 tablespoons of olive oil into a thick pan over a medium heat. Peel and slice the onion, and in the oil let it soften, not fry, for 7–10 minutes. Remove onion with a slotted spoon, add the meat, and turn it about as it lightly browns for 3–5 minutes. Remove the pan from the heat. Put the cooked onion and the raw, peeled, roughly chopped tomatoes through the Mouli, and mix with the meat in the pan. Add a little heated water or stock—¼ cup—to produce the consistency of thick soup. Add ½ a teaspoon each of sugar and salt, and a pinch each of cinnamon and nutmeg. Cook very gently without a lid for 40 minutes, adding more liquid if the mixture threatens to dry out.

Cook the macaroni until it is just done, drain, rinse in very hot water, and mix into it 1 tablespoon butter. Butter an ovenproof dish, preferably about 3 inches deep. Pour into it half the macaroni, and about a third of the grated cheese. Make an even layer of all the meat. Cover with the rest of the macaroni and more cheese. Beat the 4 eggs in a bowl with a fork and add them to the Béchamel sauce. Pour the sauce carefully over the dish, filling it almost to the top. Sprinkle over the rest of the cheese.

Put into a slow oven (325°). The top should brown lightly in about ¾ hour. The dish is then ready to serve but can remain in an oven turned very low almost indefinitely. In Greece the pasticcio is made in a rectangular dish, and served in square pieces.

26. A Simple Risotto

Many of the composite rice dishes from the countries around the Mediterranean—paella, pilaff, and so on—are too filling for the ulcer diet, and too likely to contain undercooked pieces of meat or fish.

Risotto, on the other hand, is useful. Unfortunately, it takes a full ½ hour of attention immediately before the meal, which not everyone can spare.

The authoritative description of the dish, and many delicious variations of it, some suitable for those with ulcers, are to be found in Elizabeth David, *Italian Food.* I include here only a simple one which I sometimes make to use up the stock and bits of meat left over from a baked chicken.

1½ *pints good chicken stock, free of fat*
8 *oz. cooked chicken* (*not skin or gristle*)
8 *oz. Italian rice* (*see p.* 40)
1 *stick celery, chopped fine*
1 *tablespoon olive oil*
seasonings
grated mild cheese

The quantity of chicken will be what you can pare off the skeleton, and can vary without doing any harm.

Have two adjacent burners on low. On one have the stock, keeping hot, and on the other put a thick pan, in which you will make the risotto.

Into this pan put the oil. Add first the celery, then the rice, and cook them over the low heat for 3–4 minutes only. Begin to add the hot stock a cupful at a time, at 5-minute intervals. The rice will absorb each cup of liquid in turn, so that you will have to use a wooden spoon or spatula to stop it from sticking. With the last cupful of stock, add the pieces of chicken. When this is absorbed the risotto is done. Taste and season with salt and very little pepper. The whole process will take ½ an hour but you should check to be quite sure that the rice is cooked, and, if necessary, cook a little longer. Sprinkle each helping generously with grated cheese.

27. Kedgeree

1 *lb. smoked haddock* or *other fish*
8 *oz. rice*
milk
2 *tablespoons butter*
2 *tablespoons cream*
2 *eggs*
seasonings
2 *tablespoons seedless raisins, optional*
1 *tablespoon sherry, optional*

Some ulcer diets forbid smoked fish, in which case the kedgeree can be made with any flaky white fish. So made (and without the raisins) it is the blandest and easiest of dishes to eat. But if you are allowed the smoked haddock, the result will be a more satisfying dish for a family meal.

Cook the rice (Indian if possible, see p. 40) until tender. Put it into a low oven to dry. Cover the smoked haddock with half milk, half water. Put in 6 peppercorns and a bay leaf and cook gently until it is soft (15–20 minutes). When cool enough to handle, skin it, remove all bones, and flake it. Hard boil, shell and slice the eggs. With a large fork mix the haddock, eggs and rice in a bowl that will fit into a saucepan.

Put this bowl over fast-boiling water and with the fork gradually work first the butter in pieces, then the cream into the mixture. Taste, add salt and a little pepper if needed. Cover and leave to heat through before serving.

If you include the raisins (which really must be seedless), let them warm and soften in the sherry, or in water, in the oven while the rice is drying. Add them with the fish and the eggs.

28. Haddock Soufflé

½–¾ lb. smoked haddock
3 egg yolks
4 egg whites
milk
2 tablespoons flour
2 tablespoons butter
2 tablespoons grated cheese
peppercorns
bayleaf

Just cover the haddock with milk, into which you put 6 peppercorns and a bay leaf. Cook gently until soft (about 15 minutes). Lift out the fish and strain off ⅓ pint of the milk. When the fish is cool enough, remove the skin and flake the meat.

Make a white sauce with 2 tablespoons butter and 2 of flour, for which you use the ⅓ pint of milk from the fish. When the sauce is smooth, add the flaked fish.

If you have a blender, put the mixture into it. If not, put it through the coarsest sieve of the Mouli. (I do it this way, and think it better for ulcers, but since a lot of fibre will stay behind start with more haddock: ¾ lb.)

Return to its pan, which you have rinsed and dried, warm gently, add the 3 beaten yolks and 3 oz. of some mild English cheese such as Cheddar, grated.

Add neither salt nor pepper. Leave mixture to cool. Just before the meal fold in the 4 stiffly beaten egg whites, pour into a buttered 1-pint soufflé dish and cook standing in a baking-tin of water for 30 minutes at 360°.

29. Cauliflower Cheese

1 *medium-sized cauliflower* — 1 *pint cheese sauce* (*see p.* 160)

Divide the cauliflower into sprigs. Discard the centre and cut off all hard bits of it from the stems using a sharp knife. Boil the sprigs in ¼ inch of salted water kept bubbling steadily for 10–12 minutes, but no more. Drain them well and arrange them flowers up in a shallow oven dish. Make the cheese sauce, pour it over them and put the dish into a moderate oven (350°) for 20–30 minutes, or into a hotter one (425°) for 15–20 minutes. The dish should only heat through thoroughly, not brown on top.

If you like your own recipe better than mine, use it, but don't cook and serve a cauliflower whole to an ulcer sufferer, for the fibrous centre is harmful. The cheese should be in a sauce, not just grated. Plenty of it is better for those on this diet, and nicer for everyone.

Cauliflower cheese lacks the substance to be the mainstay of any but the lightest invalid meal. In good times I prefer it, as it was once given to me in a perfectly balanced ulcer meal, as a first course, followed by plainly baked fish with rice, and then by stewed fruit and cream.

30. Stuffed Courgettes

All recipes I have ever tried for stuffing huge marrows have failed me. Unless you know one which avoids the effect of uncooked, indigestible stuffing inside raw, watery marrow, you should leave this dish out of the diet.

The young marrows, or courgettes, are quite different. The medium-sized ones, about 6 or 7 inches long, are ideal for stuffing, split open lengthways. Mixtures of meat or fish and rice, or rice, well-seasoned, alone can be used.

One of the best ways as a first course, and the perfect dish for a troubled stomach, is the Greek recipe called Little Shoes, which I have adapted below.

Little Shoes

- 1 *lb. courgettes* (2 *medium-sized ones*), *unpeeled*
- 1 *large onion*
- 2 *slices stale bread*
- 6 *oz. grated cheese* (*any mild English one*)
- 4 *peppercorns*
- *salt*
- *a small bunch of parsley*
- 2 *eggs*
- 1 *tablespoon butter*
- ¾ *pint Béchamel sauce* (*see p.* 160)

Cut the ends off the courgettes, wash them and boil them in salted water for 15 minutes. Leave in a colander to drain.

Cut up the onion and cook for 20 minutes with 4 peppercorns in just enough water to cover. Cut the crusts off the pieces of bread, then cut the slices into small pieces and add as many of these to the onion as will absorb what water is left. Put this mixture through the food mill and mix into it the butter, most of the grated cheese, chopped parsley, 1 of the eggs lightly beaten with a fork, and a teaspoon of salt.

Split the marrows lengthways and scoop out a strip in each for the stuffing. Spread this evenly into the spaces you've made and put them into a shallow oven dish.

Make the Béchamel sauce, cooking a bay leaf with it to flavour it strongly. When tepid, remove the bay leaf and add the other egg, also beaten with a fork.

Pour the sauce over the marrows, sprinkle over the remaining grated cheese and bake in a hot oven (375°–400°) until the top is barely browning, 15–25 minutes.

The dish can be prepared for the oven the morning (or even the day) before, leaving the pouring over of the sauce until nearer the cooking. It can be baked more slowly and finished under the grill, and it can be kept warm in a low oven for an hour or so without coming to any harm.

Fish

31. Poaching of fish, and trout poached in broth
32. Baked fillets of fresh haddock
33. Grilled sole
34. Sole in cream sauce
35. Fish kebabs
36. Fish croquettes
37. Steamed turbot and Hollandaise sauce
38. Cod à la Boulangère
39. Fillets of cod with sea-kale beet
40. Fish pie
41. Halibut mornay
42. Fish au gratin
43. Baked halibut with hot tomato sauce
44. Smoked haddock in cheese sauce
45. Cold baked codling
46. Mackerel with gooseberry sauce
47. Grilled herrings

INTRODUCTION

The choice and cooking of fish are subjects that stretch beyond the scope of this book, and beyond my competence. In my recipes I suggest only fish which are commonly available and which can without difficulty be prepared to serve to someone with an ulcer.

But if you like fish and have a good source of supply, you can scarcely serve it too often. No food gets such general acclamation from authorities on the care of ulcers.

There are many ways to cook fish that are acceptable: baking, poaching, grilling. They are more trouble than frying, but not much. I have given an example of each at the beginning of this section, in the forms of actual recipes rather than general directions. These can then be applied to other fish. Since ulcer sufferers should not eat the skin, I see no point in recipes which coat the outside of the fish with something, or which make it harder to see what you are eating.

Much advice given in cookery books about the buying of fish is now quite out of date. I for one would not try, with a queue shuffling behind me, to judge freshness by brilliance of eye or rosy colour of gills. Far more sensible is to find the best fish shop in your area and as long as it continues to supply you with fresh fish, to stick with it. If you find out what days the fish arrives—Friday will certainly be one of them—you can time your fish meals for these days. Experienced and devoted fish eaters have told me, and I have confirmed, that you get better results always by ordering fish in advance, and having it kept on ice from the time it arrives until you come to collect it.

The absence of a particular fish from my recipes might be wrongly taken to suggest that it is unsuited to the ulcer diet. In some cases it means no more than that I never succeeded in finding a recipe for it which I could wholeheartedly endorse.

I therefore include here a full table which will, I hope, answer the questions that are likely to arise for anyone considering a fish for a particular meal:

Brill. Excellent, regarded in recipes as interchangeable with turbot, less expensive, seldom available in many areas.

Bloaters and kippers. Not recommended by most authorities for inclusion in the ulcer diet.

Cod. See recipes.

Coley. This, the coalfish, *Gadus virens*, regarded by many as a food only for cats, is I think the best buy in fish at this moment. It is only for use in made-up dishes such as fish pie, and the fish croquettes on p. 70. It must be fresh.

Haddock. Fresh haddock costs the same as, or a little more than, cod, and some cookery and diet writers treat these as interchangeable. To me haddock has a distinct taste of its own, which you may like or not. See recipes.

Hake. Good cooked like fresh haddock.

Halibut. See recipes.

Herrings. Herrings are cheap, outstanding for nutritional value and full of flavour. They are also bony and encased in an oily skin which no ulcer sufferer should eat. See recipe on p. 79.

Mackerel. See recipe

Plaice. Much recommended for the ulcer diet by every authority, much disliked by me and every ulcer sufferer I know because we've been given it too often at bad times. If the flavour is liked in your house, and you don't object to the low proportion of meat to skin, you can serve it as often as you like and every cookery book has recipes.

Salmon and Salmon Trout. These expensive fish get a mixed but generally suspicious treatment from authorities on the ulcer diet. If absolutely fresh, and not overcooked, they seem to me just about safe; certainly not to be eaten often or except at good periods.

Sea Bass. Excellent for the ulcer diet, very rarely available.

Sea Bream. In my experience too scaly and bony to be recommended.

Shellfish. Mussels, cockles and oysters are to be avoided. Shrimps, prawns and scallops, rarely and in small quantities, are generally thought safe. Crab and lobster turn up in books on ulcer cookery but I find them upsetting and don't recommend them.

Skate. This is widely recommended, but a shortage of it coincided with my writing of this book. The recipe that looked best, with a cheese sauce, is in Elizabeth David, *French Provincial Cooking*. Do not, obviously, serve skate with black butter.

Smelts. These are precisely the kind of fish to be avoided in catering for those with ulcers: small, and with bones and skin inextricable from edible flesh.

Smoked Haddock. The ordinary smoked haddock on the bone is to be preferred to either the small fillets or the brilliantly coloured 'golden' variety which, I am told but cannot verify, is cod, and dyed as well as smoked. See recipes on pp. 57 and 76.

Sole Dover sole, though expensive, justifies its cost to those who can afford it. Little goes to waste and this fish sometimes finds favour with those who otherwise wouldn't eat anything. It is also a completely unhazardous main course for a celebration meal. I offer two recipes, more or less matching these two opposed occasions.

Tinned Fish. Surprisingly, to me, some of these are admitted by authorities into the ulcer diet: pilchards, for instance. I myself recommend only very occasionally, or when in shopping difficulties, tuna or sardines; in either case, with all bones removed, well-drained of oil on a paper towel, and well-chopped or mashed with a fork. There are some pleasant kipper pastes in jars which can also be used on such occasions.

Trout. See recipe, p. 65.

Turbot. If you want to serve a grand meal based on an expensive fish, then for someone with an ulcer turbot is a better choice than salmon. See recipe, p. 70.

Whiting. Many English people feel about its flavour as I do about that of plaice: it reminds them of illness. Otherwise, perfectly usable in the ulcer diet.

On the following page is a helpful table supplied to me by the White Fish Authority, which tells when each fish is available, and at its best. Fish, such as mackerel, which do not come within the scope of the Authority, are omitted from the table, and I could find no reliable source of up-to-date information on these.

Some books for further exploration are suggested in my bibliography.

Anyone who has not cooked fish often may find it helpful to be told that half a pound per adult is the usual quantity to buy.

31. Poaching of Fish, and Trout Poached in Broth

The cooking of fish in water is important to the ulcer diet. In practice simple and satisfactory, it requires some explanation for those new to it.

WHITE FISH	JAN.	FEB.	MAR.	APR.	MAY	JUNE	JULY	AUG.	SEPT.	OCT.	NOV.	DEC.	BEST SEASON
BASS					x	x	x	x					
BRILL	x	x	x	x	x					x	x	x	
COD	x	x	x	x	x	x	x	x	x	x	x	x	October to January
DABS	x	x	x	x	x	x	x	x	x	x	x	x	June to February
HADDOCK	x	x	x	x	x	x	x	x	x	x	x	x	June to February
HAKE	x	x	x	x	x	x	x	x	x	x	x	x	June to January
HALIBUT	x	x	x	x	x	x	x	x	x	x	x	x	July to March
PLAICE	x				x	x	x	x	x	x	x	x	
SKATE	x	x	x	x	x	x	x	x	x	x	x	x	
SOLE	x	x	x	x	x	x	x	x	x	x	x	x	July to March
TURBOT	x	x	x	x	x	x	x	x	x	x	x	x	July to March
WHITING	x	x	x	x	x	x	x	x	x	x	x	x	

Fish

1. The formidable-sounding *court bouillon* of high cookery merely exemplifies a useful discovery made by some, to me, unknown cook: that fish emerges best from poaching in water which has been previously flavoured by simmering with vegetables, herbs and seasonings.

If you are short of time you can, of course, poach in plain salted water, or put seasonings in with the fish. But, in trying all these ways, I have proved to my own satisfaction that the method described in the recipe below is the ideal one.

2. Whatever the poaching liquid, it should never boil hard but be kept at, or just below, boiling point. For once this is easy to achieve on modern cookers because the burner will only heat a small area of the cooking liquid.

3. You will need a large flat pan of some kind to poach in which will hold the fish comfortably: a large frying pan, a roasting-pan (clean, of course, not rusty or covered in baked fat), or, as I use, the lid of a large enamelled steel casserole.

Fish kettles are extremely expensive and essential only for very big fish. A rack of some kind, if you have or can get one to fit the pan, will make it much easier to lift out without breaking it.

Trout Poached in Broth

1 *or more trout*
1 *carrot*
1 *onion*
bay leaf
parsley
seasonings
for serving with the trout:
butter
lemon

Fill your poaching-pan with enough water to cover the fish—but don't put the fish into it! Put in instead a carrot and an onion, peeled and sliced, a small handful of washed parsley, 6 peppercorns, a teaspoon of salt and a small bay leaf. Bring to the boil, cook gently for $\frac{3}{4}$ hour, strain out and discard the vegetables and seasonings, keeping the flavoured water. You can prepare this broth well before you want to cook the trout.

When you are ready, bring the broth to the barest boil, slip it off the burner while you put in the trout, return it to the burner and watch to see that it does no more than tremble while the fish poaches. An average-sized trout (weighing less than 1 lb.) cooks in 25 minutes. The time will vary with the size of the fish, and a skewer inserted near the backbone will tell you when the fish is done. Lift it on to a hot plate and serve at once.

A freshly caught trout needs no accompaniment but slices of lemon and some melted butter with chopped parsley in it. Tank and farm trout are more pleasant to eat with an egg-based sauce, such as Hollandaise (p. 71). Delicate herbs like chervil and tarragon are improvements to this sauce, but with trout the best sauce I know is the Scandinavian Hollandaise with a good deal of finely chopped fresh dill added to it.

32. Baked Fillets of Fresh Haddock

The best English cook I ever knew regarded some hint of tomato as essential to the flavour of haddock, and I have followed her two ways ever since. The first is good enough to give to guests; the second is faster, cheaper, and blander.

I

½ lb. haddock fillet per person
tomatoes
mushrooms
butter
seasonings
parsley

Buy the thickest pieces of fillet the fishmonger will sell you, avoiding the tail end if possible. Get him to skin the fish if he will. Divide it into serving portions before cooking, since after it easily falls apart. For every 1 lb. of fish wash 4 small tomatoes, cut them into quarters and put them raw through the Mouli. Blend them with 2 tablespoons of butter over the lowest heat and add ¼ lb. of mushrooms, washed and sliced. Do not cook, but merely mix. Put the fillets into a buttered oven dish, spread the mushroom mixture over them, sprinkle with salt, a little grated pepper and a little finely chopped parsley. Bake in a slow to moderate oven (325°–350°) for 25–30 minutes.

II

½ lb. haddock fillet per person	*tomatoes*
white sauce (see p. 160)	

Make ¼ pint of white sauce to each ½ lb. of fish, Mouli into it 1 small washed raw tomato, pour this over the fish and bake as before.

Either way of cooking haddock is good with plain boiled rice.

33. Grilled Sole

A sole skinned and gutted but left whole is the easiest to handle. Pre-heat the grill at a half-way setting. Brush both sides of the fish lightly with oil. Grill one side for about 7 minutes, very carefully turn it over and do the other side for the same time. Check with a skewer that the fish just comes away from the backbone, and serve with slices of lemon.

34. Sole in Cream Sauce

2 Dover soles	*2 tablespoons cream, optional*
1½ oz. butter	*seasonings*
2 heaped tablespoons flour	*lemon*
8 oz. (½ pint) milk	*other ingredients as you choose*

This is a simplified version of the restaurant method of dishing up a poached sole in a cream sauce, usually with something added.

Place the skinned whole soles in a flat buttered oval oven dish and cover them with ½ pint of cold water. Add 4 peppercorns, a teaspoon of salt, a piece of lemon rind and either a bay leaf or some such fresh herbs as parsley, fennel, tarragon or chervil. Put the dish into a pre-heated oven at 350°. It will be cooked in 15 minutes, more or less.

When it has been in for 5, begin making a white sauce, taking care to cook the flour in the butter long enough to get rid of its taste—at least 3 minutes. Add the warmed milk, ½ pint if you aren't going to add cream later, about 8 oz. if you are. Cook 5–7 minutes.

Check the sole with a skewer to be sure it is cooked, and then turn the oven down to 250°. Drain almost all the liquid from the fish into a jug. Cover the fish with foil or butter paper and return it to the oven. Strain the cooking liquid and add it slowly and carefully to the white sauce. Add the 2 tablespoons of cream, if you intend to, at this stage. Simply stir it in until smooth, but don't wait for the sauce to thicken further. Drain off any liquid that remains on the fish, pour over the sauce, and serve in the same dish.

The sauce is a little dull if nothing at all is put into it. If you used fresh herbs in cooking, then the addition of more of the same—finely chopped chervil and tarragon, for instance—makes an exquisite dish.

The sauce also forms the basis of many of those Edwardian recipes, the lists of which clutter up so many cookery books. For someone with an ulcer, you won't obviously start adding lobster tails, or mussels, or oysters, though the odd, small, cooked shrimp or prawn is harmless enough.

The version called Doria is pleasant for this diet: pieces of cucumber, which were meant to be cut into little balls, but can equally well be little cubes, treated as described in the vegetable chapter (p. 124), and added, cooked, to the sauce. Alternatively, small mushrooms, barely warmed up in butter, are pleasant additions. The sauce can have grated cheese added to it.

Perhaps nicest of all to eat, certainly most tedious for the cook, is Sole Véronique, in which the dark-skinned Muscat grapes, peeled and seeded, are added to the sauce.

35. Fish Kebabs

½ lb. cod per person, as described below
bay leaves
olive oil
lemon

Buy one piece of cod steak cut from the thick part of the fish. Allow some extra weight for the bones and skin you'll remove.

Take off the skin with a very sharp knife and cut away from the backbone the two thick pieces of meat on either side. From these cut 1½–2-inch cubes of fish, and thread them on to skewers with bay leaves in between. Keep the prepared kebabs in the refrigerator until you are ready to cook them.

Get the grill extremely hot, put the kebabs carefully on to the rack, brush the top side lightly with olive oil and grill it only 3 minutes. Using a spatula, turn the kebabs over, brush the side now turned up with oil and grill it for 3 minutes. Turn the grill down to half its heat and grill for another 5 minutes.

Lift kebabs with a spatula on to hot plates, slide out the skewers (with an oven cloth, or you'll burn your fingers), and serve with lemon slices and a dish of plain boiled rice.

Often as I have watched this excellent way of cooking fish done in Greece and Turkey, I find it hard to get right at home. The fish dries if cooked too long and falls apart if handled roughly. But done well it tastes delicious, is not expensive, and could harm no stomach. Halibut or other more costly fish can be used; at the White Tower in Charlotte Street they use turbot!

36. Fish Croquettes

¾ lb. inexpensive white fish
2 slices day-old French bread
1 egg
seasonings
crisp toasted breadcrumbs
parsley
a sauce (see below)

Get the fishmonger to skin the fish, or do it yourself, and remove the bones. Put it raw through the mincer. Cut the crusts off the bread and soak the slices in a little milk. When soft, squeeze out the soaked bread with your fingers and using them blend bread, minced fish, egg, salt and a very little pepper, and a tablespoon of finely chopped parsley. Form into 2-inch balls, roll in the breadcrumbs and steam for 20 minutes. Lift out on to a hot plate and pour over ½ a pint of white sauce, to which you have added either a fresh tomato put raw through the Mouli, or more chopped parsley, or both.

This quantity of fish croquettes will just fit on to the vegetable steaming rack (described on p. 116) and will feed two people. A larger quantity poses problems of cooking which should be considered before you start.

These are prepared in under 15 minutes, including washing-up the mincer. They are light and pleasant to eat and can be made with any white fish, including coley, in which case the dish is extremely cheap.

37. Steamed Turbot and Hollandaise Sauce

When you pay so much, a simple cooking method seems sensible, to preserve the texture and not to confuse the taste of the turbot. A steamer such as the one described in the vegetable section does the job well, but you must have a pan big enough to hold the piece of turbot sitting on the rack.

If you lack the equipment for steaming, an equally good method is to cook the fish in a prepared broth, as explained on p. 65.

Cooking time for poaching in broth is about 10 minutes per pound; for steaming, nearer 15. In either case a touch with a skewer will tell you when the fish will just part from its bone, and is therefore cooked. The bigger the piece of turbot, the better it will taste and the more evenly it will cook.

A small heated jug filled with melted butter, and slices of lemon are good accompaniments. For a festive occasion a Hollandaise sauce suits turbot well. The recipe follows.

Hollandaise Sauce

3 *egg yolks*	1 *dessertspoon lemon juice*
6 *oz. butter*	*salt*

This quantity of sauce accompanies 2 lb. of fish, for 4 people.

Into a bowl which will fit into a saucepan put the yolks, beat them well with a fork, add the lemon juice, a little salt and beat again. Put the bowl into the pan over water which is scarcely boiling and begin to add the butter, a teaspoon at a time. Stir in each new piece until the sauce has smoothed and thickened again. When all the butter is added the sauce is done. Taste to see if it needs more salt, or a drop or two more of lemon juice.

If the water boils hard, the yolks will scramble. If you turn off the heat and leave the sauce over the water it will keep warm and survive while you serve the meal. But it will not keep forever and is most difficult to re-heat without spoiling. This moment of assembling people while the sauce waits is the tricky one, making it is not troublesome.

Some blenders have their own method of making Hollandaise, which their instructions describe. It is said to be foolproof. Many cookery writers have theories, also said to be foolproof. Follow any recipe you like the sound of but not those containing vinegar, onions or shallots.

38. Cod à la Boulangère (Adapted from *Madame Prunier's Fish Cookery Book*)

2 thick cod steaks, together weighing about 1 lb.
1 lb. potatoes
1 small onion
2 tablespoons butter
parsley

Remove all skin from the pieces of fish, either by dipping the edge in boiling water or simply with a sharp knife.

Peel the onion very carefully, removing all papery skin and tough outer spheres; peel potatoes. Put them together, whole, into cold water. Bring to the boil and cook for 15 minutes. Drain, quarter, place around the fish in a buttered shallow oven dish. Pour over the melted butter.

Bake for 35–40 minutes at 375°. Half way through the cooking, take out the dish and baste fish and vegetables with butter. Sprinkle with chopped parsley and serve.

At the right time of year, new potatoes and small onions can be used, when they will require only 10 minutes preboiling, and no quartering.

Serve without onions to the ulcer sufferer.

39. Fillets of Cod with Seakale Beet

1 lb. thick fillets of cod
stems only from 1 plant of seakale beet
thick cheese sauce (*see p.* 160)

Place the cod fillets skin down in a broad bowl and pour in ¼ inch boiling water. Peel off the skin (if the fillets aren't thick this proves impossible).

Cook the stems for 1 hour as described on p. 129. Place the skinned cod fillets on top of the stems, pour over the cheese sauce and cook uncovered at 325° for 25–30 minutes.

You can also use hake, or any white fish.

40. Fish Pie

1½ *lb. skinned fillets of cod, coley* or *other white fish*	½ *pint milk*
3 *eggs*	*butter*
4 *small tomatoes*	*flour*
½ *lb. small mushrooms*	*parsley*
1½ *lb. potatoes*	*seasonings*

The recipe involves getting ingredients ready, then building up the pie and re-heating it.

To prepare ingredients:

1. Cook the fish in ½ pint milk in a wide shallow pan with 1 teaspoon salt, 6 peppercorns, a bay leaf and a blade of mace for only 5–10 minutes, until it will just flake.
2. Boil the eggs for 8 minutes, plunge them into cold water and peel them.
3. Pour boiling water over the tomatoes and peel them.
4. Melt 2 tablespoons of butter, take this off the heat, turn the well-washed mushrooms about in it and leave them to absorb it.
5. Cook the potatoes and make a purée, your own way or mine (123).
6. Strain the milk in which the fish has cooked and make a white sauce using 3 tablespoons butter and 2 tablespoons flour.

Then:

1. Flake the fish, removing all bones, and put into the

bottom of a soufflé dish or earthenware casserole holding 3 pints.

2. Scatter over the chopped parsley.
3. Pour over the white sauce.
4. Arrange the mushrooms in an even layer.
5. Pour over half the potato purée.
6. Slice in first the eggs, then the tomatoes.
7. Pour over the rest of the purée.

If you like, decorate the top with 2 oz. of the cooked peeled shrimps fishmongers sell. Reheat the dish at 300° for ¾–1 hour, covered with foil or a lid, in a pan of water.

This dish makes a mountain of washing-up but it can be prepared as much as a day in advance and kept warm (at a slightly lower oven setting) for a long time on the day you eat it.

41. Halibut Mornay

1 lb. halibut
2 lb. potatoes
milk
butter
flour
1 egg
6 tablespoons grated mild cheese

Peel the potatoes and put them on to boil. Meanwhile, make ¾ pint of cheese sauce, by your own method or the one on p. 160.

Likewise, by your way or the one on p. 123 make a purée of the potatoes. Steam the halibut or poach it in just simmering salted water only until it will come off the bone (5–10 minutes).

Choose a flat ovenproof dish which you can see will be filled by the ingredients. Butter it. Add to the potatoes, off the burner, an egg which you have beaten in a bowl with a fork. Do not wash bowl or fork.

By holding the ovenproof dish in one hand and spooning

with the other, make an even ring of the potatoes, leaving a hole in the middle. With the egg fork, and what little egg remains in the bowl, make a criss-cross pattern on the potatoes. Pour a very little of the cheese sauce into the middle of the dish, then the fish, free of bones and skin, in the large flakes into which it naturally falls as you handle it. Pour the remaining cheese sauce into the middle of the dish only, so that a ring of patterned potatoes remains standing around the outside.

Either straightaway, or later if it suits you, put the dish into a hot oven (400°) for about 15 minutes and bring it out when the potatoes are barely beginning to brown. Don't leave it longer, or the fish will overcook and the cheese sauce form a hard crust, which is bad for the ulcer sufferer.

42. Fish au Gratin

1 *lb. any white fish*	*other ingredients as in preceding recipe*

Halibut Mornay is a restaurant dish, easy to produce at home, impressive-looking and delicious. The combination of white fish, sauce and potatoes is ideal for the ulcer diet and, as any cook will realize, can be much varied. It can be made with other white fish, including the less expensive ones; but cod, for instance, needs light handling if it is not to turn into a stringy mess. It, or any other fish, needs only minimal cooking before flaking, since it cooks more as the dish is warmed in the oven. Restaurants make the dish with fillets of white fish, skinned and rolled; but this, too, obviously takes some skill in preparation.

Parsley sauce can be used instead of cheese. A scattering of 3 tablespoons of roasted breadcrumbs looks pretty and makes the dish officially *au gratin*. Whatever the variation, care is needed not to toast the top of the dish into a hard crust.

43. Baked Halibut with Hot Tomato Sauce

This recipe is adapted from one in André Simon's *Guide to Good Food and Wine* (see Bibliography). It is easy, quite quick, and produces the best results I have had with halibut.

1 lb. halibut
6 small or *4 medium tomatoes*
half a lemon
½ pint milk
1 tablespoon butter
seasonings

Remove the dark skin by dipping that side of the fish into boiling water, or pouring it carefully from a kettle over the side until the skin peels away neatly.

Place fish in a casserole. Add enough milk to come half way up the fish, salt and 6 peppercorns. Bake gently (oven 300°–325°), basting once or twice.

Once the fish is cooking slice the washed but unpeeled tomatoes into quarters. Melt the butter gently in a small pan, put in the pieces of tomato, squeeze the lemon and drop it in too, just as it is. Stew gently until the fish is nearly done (you can put it into an oven dish on the bottom shelf while the fish is cooking if you like). Then put the whole mixture through the Mouli, which will leave behind lemon peel, skin and seeds of tomato. Keep hot.

Test the fish after ¾ hour to see if it is cooked. When it is, lift it out carefully on to a heated plate. Pour the sauce over or serve it separately in a small heated jug.

44. Smoked Haddock in Cheese Sauce

½ lb. smoked haddock per person
¼ pint white sauce per person (*see p.* 160)
2 tablespoons mild English cheese, grated
seasonings
hard-boiled eggs

For a meal in a hurry, smoked haddock can simply be simmered for 10–15 minutes in ⅔ milk, ⅓ water, with a small bay leaf and 4 peppercorns. But this dish, a standby of English households during postwar meat shortages, is little more trouble, filling and generally satisfactory.

Cook the haddock as just described and take the flesh carefully away from bones and skin. To the heated white sauce add the cheese and, when it melts, the flaked haddock and some sliced hard-boiled eggs. Heat through and serve, or put into an oven dish and heat when required. Serve with rice, or for a simple supper, on toast.

See also the soufflé of smoked haddock on p. 54.

45. Cold Baked Codling

For a large family, or a party of six or more people, I know nothing that costs so little, tastes so good, or looks so welcoming on the table as this. To do it you must have a co-operative fishmonger, a roll of the wide (20-inch) kitchen foil and a long plate to serve the fish on—18 inches or more.

Ask the fishmonger a day or two before you want the fish to get for you specially a codling—a whole young cod—weighing 5 lb. or less. If you have a small cooker measure your oven and give him a maximum length. Ask him to clean out the insides from the fish, but leave head and tail intact.

The sooner you collect the fish and cook it, the better; obviously it is better eaten the same day, too. Cooked, it can be kept in the refrigerator for one day.

Measure the right length of foil, leaving 6 inches over for the ends. Oil it well and put the fish on to it.

Chop together parsley and any other fresh herb you can get: fennel, dill, chervil, tarragon. Dried herbs should work well enough, too. Stuff the herbs into the fish, squeeze over the juice of $\frac{1}{2}$ a lemon and sprinkle on some salt. Very carefully seal the fish into the foil. If necessary use another length on top to make the foil secure.

Pre-heat a low oven—300°—for 10 minutes, then put in the fish and cook if for a full 25 minutes per pound. At the end of the cooking, open the oven door and let the fish cool down on the rack. Then with extreme care undo the foil and lift the fish on to its plate.

Surround if you like by small cold new potatoes as described on p. 139; at any rate serve it with a well-thinned mayonnaise.

I'm told a codling cooked this way is also good hot.

46. Mackerel with Gooseberry Sauce

for 2 mackerel:
½ *lb.* (or 1 *tin*) *gooseberries*
2 *oz. butter*
1 *level tablespoon flour*
seasonings

This famous combination of fish and fruit is too good to miss. But undiluted gooseberries are too fierce for a tender stomach so they must be made into a simple sauce.

Either grill the mackerel, cleaned, brushed with oil and lemon juice, for 10–15 minutes; or, I think better, poach them in a broth as described on p. 65, with the addition of the juice of ½ a lemon, for about 25–30 minutes.

The gooseberries, if fresh, can be stewed in very little water without topping and tailing, sweetened well, and put through the Mouli; tinned ones simply put through the Mouli. Keep separately either the cooking juice or the liquid from the tin. Measure ½ a cup (5 fl. oz.) of this and put it on to heat.

Blend the flour with the butter over a gentle heat and cook a full 5 minutes. Add first the heated juice and then, when it is blended, the gooseberry purée. Add salt, a sprinkling of nutmeg, cook for 5 minutes and it is ready. If it gets too thick waiting for the fish to be cooked, add a little more of the juice to it.

47. Grilled Herrings

2 herrings per person | *lemons*
cooking oil

After a two-year search through cookery books, much trial and error, advice sought and unsought from friends, and encouragement from the helpful Herring Industry Board, I conclude that the best way to include herrings in this book is plain grilled, with two fish for every adult.

The last is important. Some waste should be positively encouraged (as the only alternative to eating skin and bones) and enough fish provided to make this possible. Additions such as oatmeal make it harder to see what you are doing when you eat the fish. Finally, herrings are a choice to celebrate a good period, not an invalid dish.

Some fishmongers, but not all, will bone or scale herrings. You can learn to do this yourself, but I no longer do. I simply wash the cleaned and beheaded herrings in salt water, and dry them in a kitchen paper towel.

Make three deep cuts in the side of each fish. Brush them lightly with cooking oil. Put them close to a very hot grill. They cook quickly. Turn them only once, allowing 5–7 minutes for each side. Serve them instantly with slices of lemon. Bones and skin are easy to discard on the plate. Vegetables are best served afterwards, on clean plates.

Do not serve mustard sauce to an ulcer sufferer.

Main Dishes

48. Boiled chicken
49. Baked chicken
50. Casserole of frozen chicken
51. Creamed chicken or turkey
52. Chicken cooked in milk
53. Pish-Pash
54. Roast duck, goose and turkey
55. Veal recipes in brief
56. Blanquette de veau
57. Rabbit with lentil purée
58. Best end of neck of lamb in stock
59. Roast leg of lamb
60. Shoulder of lamb with vegetables
61. Mild moussaka
62. Grilling of meat
63. Baked chops
64. Baked lamb cutlets
65. Navarin printanier
66. Skewered lamb
67. Skewered liver and bacon
68. Ham in white sauce
69. Boiled beef
70. Meat loaf
71. Hamburgers
72. Braised beef with summer vegetables
73. Stewed shin of beef

Tender steak, lamb or veal chops, plainly grilled, are most frequently recommended as ulcer fare. When the budget will stand them, they certainly do save the cook's time, and are pleasant and safe for any ulcer sufferer to eat. Directions for grilling meat are given on p. 98.

Most of my suggestions are for generally much cheaper dishes, to feed a number of people, and often include their own vegetables. Many of them involve forethought and advance preparation. These have the great advantage that, if you have done your work in good time, you won't run the risk of serving the meal late.

You'd have to go out of your way to make a chicken upsetting to an ulcer sufferer. Unless you fry it, curry it, or add some forbidden ingredient to it, you can cook it as you like: slowly in a casserole, fast under a grill, with any of the many herbs that suit it, roast with stuffing or without, whole or jointed, served hot or cold, in rice or on it, and so on.

Cookery writers agree that $\frac{1}{4}$ lb. of meat is the correct amount to allow for each adult. This means lean meat. In buying poultry, or joints with bones and skin which won't be eaten, due allowance must be made for the waste.

48. Boiled Chicken

a large boiling fowl
2 *large carrots*
2 *onions*
2 *leeks, when available*
2 *pieces celery, when available*
parsley
seasonings

This group of vegetables is I think the ideal one, but when leeks or celery are not available some others, such as small turnips, can be substituted.

Into a thick pot big enough to hold everything comfortably put the chicken and its giblets (to flavour the chicken, not for eating), both washed in cold water. Add the peeled carrots and onions, the celery, the leeks split and carefully washed, the parsley, salt, peppercorns and a bay leaf.

Pour into the pot boiling water enough just to cover the chicken. Turn the heat under the pot on full, to bring back quickly to the boil. As it boils, skim, and continue until no scum rises. Put on the lid and turn down the heat until the water just simmers. Cook for two or three hours.

Do not serve the vegetables cooked in the pot but use more of these same vegetables plus a couple of potatoes, all boiled or, much better, steamed together (see p. 116).

The vinaigrette sauce which recipes usually recommend with this dish is not, of course, suitable for ulcers; the sauces thickened with eggs or cream at the last moment may give ulcers to the cook. So I just strain off some of the juice, skim off it what fat I can, and serve it in a heated jug.

For a way to use up the remains of this dish, see p. 85.

49. Baked Chicken

1 *roasting chicken* (3–4 *lb.*)	*salt*
3 *tablespoons oil*	*pepper*

Put the oil into a pot which is big enough to hold the chicken and which can be used on top as well as in the oven. Warm it over a low heat, put in the chicken and turn it about until the outside is very lightly browned. Put it into a low oven (310°) and cook for $1\frac{1}{2}$ hours. Turn the chicken over several times in the cooking.

50. Casserole of Frozen Chicken

Whole frozen chickens need no special treatment for the ulcer diet, except to be sure that they are fully thawed. The frozen chicken joints widely sold in this country require something extra, for they should not be fried and the instructions for grilling on many of their packets leave them not merely raw, but still frozen. They don't taste of much, either, and my reason for including them is that they may, when you are dependent upon a frozen food counter, be your only recourse.

Slow cooking in a casserole with other ingredients is undoubtedly the best way to treat them. The recipe I give is for a fancy dish for a celebratory meal, such as restaurants serve under names like *chasseur*. For ordinary occasions, or difficult periods, the method can be simpler: the onions cooked, as directed but without the tomatoes; the chicken browned, with or without the bacon; and carrots included, or peeled new potatoes added an hour before the end, instead of mushrooms. Joints of a boiling fowl can be cooked this way, or a whole frozen chicken which you cut up yourself, and with ingredients increased accordingly.

2 *joints of frozen chicken (about* 1 *lb. together)*
$\frac{1}{4}$ *lb. cheapest bacon*
$\frac{3}{4}$ *lb. mushrooms*
1 *small onion*
2 *small tomatoes*
2 *sticks celery*
$\frac{1}{2}$ *cup stock* or *water*
flour and seasonings
oil
butter

Peel and roughly slice the onion. In one dessertspoon of olive oil let it soften on a medium heat for 5 minutes. Add the peeled, roughly chopped tomatoes and $\frac{1}{2}$ cup hot water or stock. Cook 20–30 minutes and put through the Mouli.

In a thick frying pan over the same heat put a dessertspoon of oil and the bacon cut into small squares; when the fat starts to run put in the chicken pieces, first dipped in flour and salt. Turn them about to brown very lightly, for 5 minutes, no more. Remove chicken and bacon to a casserole, pour into the pan the onion and tomato mixture and scrape up flour from the pan, adding another tablespoon of water if necessary. Put the sliced celery around the chicken and pour over the mixture. Put a branch of thyme or a bay leaf on top.

Cook for 1½ hours at oven 300°. Near the end, coat the washed and sliced mushrooms with melted butter. Remove the thyme or bay leaf and put the mushrooms on top of the other ingredients in the casserole. In 10 minutes scatter a little finely chopped parsley on top and serve.

51. Creamed Chicken or Turkey

leftovers of cooked chicken or *turkey*
2 *tablespoons breadcrumbs*
6 *tablespoons grated Cheddar* or *other mild English cheese*
½ *pint milk*
4 *tablespoons cream*
2 *heaped tablespoons flour*
butter
seasonings

Pare the remains off a cooked chicken or turkey. About ½ lb., or a little over, is the quantity this recipe requires. Remove all skin, bone and gristle before weighing and then cut into pieces the same size.

Make a white sauce by adding the flour to 2 oz. butter on a low heat, cooking gently and adding gradually, off the burner, the warmed milk, stirring all the time. Return to the burner and keep stirring until it begins to thicken. Then add 2 tablespoons of stock from the bird if you have it (if not, increase the quantity of milk you start with); add the cream, a little salt, a little grated pepper, a little grated nutmeg and 4 tablespoons of the grated cheese.

Select a flat lidless oven-proof dish holding about 1 pint. Into this pour a little of the sauce. Arrange over it the pieces of meat evenly, and pour over the remaining sauce. Mix the remaining 2 tablespoons of cheese with the breadcrumbs, make an even layer of these and dot the top with a very little butter.

Put the dish on a baking-sheet in a moderate oven—370°—and cook 15–20 minutes. Near the end of the cooking put on the grill and when it is hot take the dish out of the oven and put under the grill for only 2 minutes or less, so that the top barely browns.

A dish of Italian rice, boiled, drained and put on the floor of the oven to dry as the dish cooks, goes perfectly with it.

52. Chicken Cooked in Milk

a boiling fowl, or *joints of one*
rice
milk
onions
seasonings

You can use for this dish the joints of boiling fowl which are so very cheap to buy. For two such joints, weighing 1½–2 lb. together, you will want ½ cup (¼ pint) of Italian rice, 2 onions, a small bay leaf and, finally, 4 peppercorns and some whole mace or chunks of nutmeg, in a tea infuser or tied into cheesecloth.

Put the joints into an oven dish with a cover that fits well. Wash the rice in a strainer and put it in too, then the seasonings, 2 teaspoons salt and 1 pint of milk. Peel the onions and slice them thickly on top. Cover with foil as well as the lid and cook in the lowest oven (250°) for 5–6 hours. Check once to see if more milk is needed. When you serve, take out the seasonings and bay leaf and *remove all the onions from the ulcer sufferer's portion.* Scatter finely chopped parsley over the dish.

A whole boiling fowl cooked in this way takes all day, from after breakfast until the evening. The quantities are 2 pints of milk, 1 cup of rice and a proportionate increase of onions and seasonings.

This dish is soothing but not bland, to be used in good times rather than bad; for the rice, which has absorbed all the milk and a good deal of chicken juice and fat, is really quite rich. The removal of the onions is important; those without ulcers can, of course, eat them, and will enjoy them.

53. Pish-Pash

1 *large roasting chicken*
1 *lb. basmatti rice* (*see p. 40*)
1 *large onion*
2 *small pieces whole dried ginger*
6 *corns whole allspice*
2 *tablespoons butter*
4 *bay leaves*
salt, and 6 *peppercorns*

Buy the chicken already cut up if you can. Otherwise do this yourself. Wash the rice well in a sieve. Peel the onion and slice finely. Put all these into a thick pan, add 1 teaspoon salt and the spices and seasonings and just cover with cold water. Bring to the boil, then turn down and simmer for 2 hours, or put into a low oven (300°) for this time. Fifteen minutes before serving, remove the bay leaves and spices and stir in the butter.

This is an invalid dish from India, easy, not too highly seasoned for the ulcer diet, nor too dull for other people. Children liked it when I gave it to them at a family meal, served with a dish of yoghourt. An appropriate chutney, though it must certainly not be offered to the person with ulcers, makes the dish more interesting for the others.

Whole dried ginger is easy to get, as are the whole all-spice corns. To hold these and the peppercorns (in this and other slow-cooking dishes) a small tea infuser is convenient.

Serve without onions to the person with the ulcer.

54. Roast Duck, Goose and Turkey

Domestic poultry in general suits the ulcer diet. Fat birds like duck and goose shouldn't turn up every day—and at their price they obviously won't! Turkeys can be eaten as often as you like, and the small ones weighing seven pounds or less give good value in lean meat.

Recipes as such wouldn't seem to me helpful, so I merely make suggestions for the simple cooking of each. Stuffings based on breadcrumbs or fruit are better than those containing sausage meat. The oven readings and times I give below can be no more than general guides. Your cooker may well have its own chart or book of instructions to follow; when roasting for someone with an ulcer, longer cooking at a lower temperature is always to be preferred to the faster, hotter method.

Duck

A rack in the roasting-pan is important so that the duck won't stew in its fat. A low to moderate temperature (330°–350°) for about 25 minutes per pound is best. After the first half hour the fat in the pan should be poured off and a stock made from the giblets poured in. Many good recipes exist for turning this into a sauce and for accompaniments.

I'm prejudiced against ducks for eating at home because they contain so little meat. The portions are always disappointing, which no one, but least of all someone with an ulcer, enjoys.

Goose

The rack in the pan is even more important. The oven temperature should again be low (330°), the timing up to 2½–3 hours, depending on the size of the goose. The bird should be covered with foil, which is removed for the last hour and the oven turned down to 300°. The fat should be poured off often during the cooking.

Goose seems to me both more appealing, and better for delicate stomachs, if served cold and not stuffed.

I should record that the old books on ulcer diets warned particularly against large, elderly, tough geese. The ones I can buy weigh only about 6–7 lb. and aren't tough; but should you be offered the others you should obviously refuse them.

Turkey
I have the best results by far with the small unfrozen turkeys which some good shops sell. Unlike ducks and geese they need a little olive oil, or butter, or both, rubbed over them before roasting; otherwise, they too sit on a rack, covered in foil, for 20 minutes per pound plus a further 20, at 350°. The foil is removed for the last half hour to brown the breast.

55. Veal Recipes in Brief

Although veal is excellent meat for someone with an ulcer, it is extremely expensive. The supply, outside London and some other big cities, is scarce, erratic, and to say the least variable in quality. Therefore, rather than take up space in a short book with a lot of recipes which may prove useless, I summarize briefly my experience of the various ways of treating veal, and their uses in this diet:

Escalope
Fried, this is wrong for an ulcer; grilled it is in my view a waste of expensive material.

Breast of Veal
This should not be served to someone with an ulcer.

Veal Chops
Though expensive they are good and safe and are best baked —either as described for lamb chops on p. 99; or browned under the grill and cooked more slowly in the oven with a little stock in the pan; or according to the instructions that come with your cooker.

Roast Veal
If you live where they are available, and can afford them, those exquisite little pieces of veal cut in the French way

are delicious and could do no harm to any stomach. The conventional English cut for roasting, though equally safe, is almost always dry and disappointing. Both are better done in a thick pan with a lid in a slow oven and both require longer cooking than beef or lamb. It is best to consult the instructions for your own cooker.

Shoulder and other stewing cuts

Lean shoulder meat is the only one to be recommended and the right recipe is certainly that for Blanquette de Veau, below.

Most other stewing recipes depend upon the meat's cooking in a sharp tomato sauce which breaks up the tough fibres, and then, when you eat it, does the same to your stomach.

A rolled shoulder, in the unlikely event that you find it, can be cooked like a shoulder of lamb, slowly, in a covered pan, with stock, potatoes or other vegetables.

Minced Veal

Bought from a reliable source minced veal seldom contains anything upsetting and can be grilled like minced beef (see Hamburgers, p. 104).

56. Blanquette de Veau

This is the best recipe I know for the ulcer diet. It is easy but involves a tense last 5 minutes before serving.

Breast of veal is unsuitable for this or any other dish to be given to someone with an ulcer. Shoulder or some other reasonably lean cut will do, and it is better—and quite easy—to cut it up yourself rather than having the butcher do it.

1 *lb. stewing veal* (*see paragraph above*)
1 *onion*
1 *large carrot* or 2 *small*
a piece of celery
1½ *tablespoons butter*
1½ *tablespoons flour*
4 *oz. small mushrooms*

1 *egg yolk*	1½ *tablespoons cream*
juice of ½ lemon	*herbs, spices, salt*

Cut the meat into pieces about 2 inches square, removing all skin and gristle and most fat. Put into a pan with 1 pint of water, the onion and carrot, peeled and cut up, the celery, a dessertspoon of salt, 2 cloves, 6 peppercorns, and herbs, fresh or dried: parsley, tarragon, marjoram, thyme, bay leaf, or the best selection you can get. Bring barely to the boil and simmer for 1–1¼ hours.

Strain the stock from this pan, take out the pieces of veal and keep them covered in a bowl, discard the vegetables and herbs, put the stock back in its pan and keep it boiling to reduce a little.

Blend the flour into the butter over a low heat, take off the burner and add slowly ½ pint of the hot stock (there should not be much more by now). When smooth, add the whole mushrooms, washed and minus their stalks, and simmer for ¾ hour. Beat the lemon juice and egg yolk together with a fork, add them to the mixture off the burner, add the cream, then the pieces of veal.

Return to the burner turned low and stir as it heats through. It must not boil and must be eaten the moment it is ready.

Scatter it with chopped parsley and serve with a bowl of patna rice: this is best cooked before and left drying in a low oven while you do the slightly tricky last-minute work on the *blanquette*.

57. Rabbit with Lentil Purée

1 *rabbit, jointed*	*salt*
4 *oz. lentils*	*herbs*
1 *small onion*	*butter*
1 *stick celery*	*flour*
1 *rasher of bacon*	*a little cream* or *top of milk*

Please see the general remarks about rabbit on p. 41.

For this recipe you can if you prefer buy the joints separately, choosing the meatier ones. If you want the rabbit to taste less of rabbit you can soak it in salted water; if not, just wash the pieces.

Put them, the washed lentils, peeled and sliced onion, celery, rasher of bacon, a dessertspoon of salt, 6 peppercorns, and the best bundle of herbs you can manage (or some dried ones) into a very large pan that will hold all comfortably. Put in enough water so that nothing is left uncovered. Simmer over the lowest heat, or in a low oven (325°) for about 3 hours, or until the lentils are soft and the meat tender.

Take out the pieces of rabbit and scrape off any lentils that cling to them. Strain the water off the vegetables and lentils and keep it to hand. Put the vegetables and lentils through the Mouli, a slow job. Add to them enough of the liquid to achieve the consistency of thin cream soup. In a thick pan over a low fire blend 2 tablespoons of flour and 3 of butter, and off the fire gradually add the purée. Cook it gently for 10 minutes and taste, adding salt if necessary, and a little more butter.

Just before serving add a tablespoon of cream or the top off a bottle of milk. Put the pieces back into the sauce, spoon it over them, heat through gently and serve. The dish can be kept warm in a low oven.

This dish turns up in many cookery books, with variations which may be useful to know:

1. The rabbit can be stewed alone with herbs and vegetables and some of its liquid added to a purée of lentils made separately.

2. Instead of lentils dried or fresh peas, or a mixture of vegetables such as broad beans, leeks and potatoes, are suggested for the purée.

3. If you haven't time for the complications of this recipe

you can stew the rabbit in the ordinary way with onions, carrots, herbs and seasonings and, if you like, thicken the liquid with a flour and butter mixture; if your own diet doesn't forbid it you can brown the pieces of rabbit before stewing, in oil, or a mixture of oil and butter.

58. Best End of Neck of Lamb in Stock

The ideal joint for four people—and the gentlest of food—is a best end of neck of lamb, consisting of eight cutlets; the butcher will prepare it for you by cutting through the bones so that the cutlets are left joined together, and by removing most of the fat. He will give you the long bone he removes, and other trimmings, if you ask.

From these, a sliced onion, a carrot, a handful of washed parsley, peppercorns and a bay leaf make about ½ pint of stock. Strain this and pour it over the lamb in a roasting-dish, cover with a buttered foil and cook for 1¼–1½ hours at 360°–375°, basting two or three times. Should you have a tablespoon or two of red wine you can mix it with a correspondingly reduced quantity of the stock and use this as the cooking liquid. If you want the top of the lamb to brown a little, remove the foil for the last 10–15 minutes of cooking.

The joint cuts quickly and easily into cutlets and so, unlike some roasts, is still hot when you eat it.

59. Roast Leg of Lamb

A small leg of lamb roasted with care is a good dish for someone with an ulcer. If not done properly, it can be the worst.

The way not to do it is to fill an old blackened roasting-pan half way up with fat, bring it to the sizzling point in a very hot oven and then put in the lamb surrounded by potatoes. Called roasting, this method is in effect deep-frying, and although the result is traditional and looks attractive, it will almost certainly upset a susceptible stomach.

The right way is to follow the directions given now with most new cookers for the alternative lower-temperature, slower method. If you don't have these directions you will probably find that a reading of 360°–375°, and a time of 30 minutes per pound, will be correct. But you will need to be prepared to alter time or temperature slightly; and having established these for your own oven you will be sensible, if you have a memory like mine, to write them down for future reference.

Here are other points I've found helpful in roasting lamb for myself and others with ulcers:

1. Olive oil is the best lubricant to use when roasting, but marinading in this or anything else is not to be recommended.

2. If you want to use garlic, put it whole, peeled, in the pan and take it out before serving. Don't insert slivers into the joint. Similarly, if you use rosemary, put pieces of it in the pan and not on top of the joint where spikes may get left behind.

3. Don't cook roast potatoes with the lamb. They aren't good for an ulcer sufferer and at the recommended low temperature they won't be a success anyway.

4. Use a clean roasting pan. Get a trivet or rack for the lamb to rest on, up out of the fat on the bottom.

5. Halfway through the cooking pour off most of the fat in the pan; or, if you like, pour it all away and pour over the joint a cup of good chicken stock.

6. A shoulder of lamb, if you know it to be young and tender, can be treated like this, but in general I have better results cooking it with vegetables as recommended next.

60. Shoulder of Lamb with Vegetables

This cut of meat is a great standby for the ulcer diet. Nothing from the butcher is cheap but this provides good lean meat for much less money than leg, chops or cutlets. The really cheap cuts, such as breast, are too full of fat and gristle to be suitable for the ulcer diet.

Given notice, most butchers will bone and roll a shoulder. It looks neater and is easier to slice. But the joint with the bone still in it is perfectly presentable, and perhaps keeps its flavour better. If a whole shoulder is too large for you, you can buy a half (and in the following recipes, halve the other ingredients accordingly).

Either you or the butcher should remove before cooking any excess fat you can cut off without ruining the look of the joint.

A shoulder can be roasted like a leg. If boned, it can be stuffed, which will make it go further. But I, and most people with stomachs like mine, find a shoulder cooked slowly in stock the most soothing and welcome dish in the world.

I give two seasonal variations of this way of cooking it. Anyone who cares to look through some of the cookery books I list on p. 175 will find more. You can alter the vegetables used if, for instance, you cook for a family that hates turnips. The principle of the dish remains the same.

Spring version:

a shoulder of lamb
2 bunches spring carrots
1 bunch new turnips or
2 lb. new potatoes
herbs
seasonings
butter
flour

Into a thick pan with a lid put 2 tablespoons of butter. In this, very lightly brown the side of the shoulder covered in skin; do not let the butter burn. Turn the meat over, dust a little flour into the butter and blend them. Add 4 cups of hot stock. (You can make this by boiling up the bone or trimmings or, at a pinch, just use water.)

Add salt, a bay leaf, peppercorns, marjoram, thyme and the well-scraped carrots. Put on the lid and cook at the lowest heat on top, or in a low oven (310°–325°) for 2 hours.

About ½ hour before serving, peel and quarter the turnips. Boil them for 5 minutes, drain them completely and into their pan put a tablespoon of butter. Turn them about in it over a low heat as it melts. Add them to the meat.

Test them with a skewer to be sure they are soft. When they are, skim what fat you can off the stock and serve.

If you use potatoes instead of turnips don't cut them up or pre-boil them but do coat them with butter over a low heat before adding them.

If you like, a small clove of garlic can be put into the pan with the vegetables, and removed before serving.

Winter version:

Instead of the spring vegetables use 1 small onion and 1 lb. carrots and with them a selection of leeks, turnips or swedes (but not both), celery, or whatever is available.

Prepare them in the usual way, taking care to remove the outer sphere of the onion. Cut them into fairly large pieces of about the same size and put them in at the beginning of the cooking.

With either version, serve slices of fresh bread to mop up the juice, and redcurrant jelly if you like it.

61. Mild Moussaka

As well as the famous dish made with aubergines the Greeks themselves do a lighter version which is better for the likes of us. It is a convenient way to use up the remains of a joint, particularly of lamb or mutton which are not so inviting when cold.

1 *lb. minced lamb* or *mutton* (or *any cooked meat*)
1 *onion*
1 *lb. courgettes* (*small marrows*)
2–3 *tomatoes*
olive oil
seasonings
1 *pint Béchamel sauce* (*see p.* 160)
1 *egg*

Cut the ends off the courgettes, wash them, slice them about $\frac{3}{4}$ inch thick, put them in a colander with plenty of salt and leave them for an hour or more.

Peel the onion, quarter it and simmer it in very little water for 15 minutes. Put the meat through the mincer, leaving out all skin, fat and gristle. Pour boiling water over the tomatoes then put them and the cooked onion through the food mill. Mix vegetables and meat together in a bowl, adding 1 tablespoon of oil, salt, a little pepper.

Run cold water over the courgettes in the colander, boil them steadily for 10 minutes, lift them from their pan back into the colander to drain. Empty the pan and put into it 2 tablespoons of oil. Warm this, take it off the burner. Dip each piece of courgette into it and use half of them to cover the bottom of a well-oiled casserole.

Put the meat over this in an even layer. Dip the rest of the courgettes in oil and make another layer on top of the meat. Put into a low oven (325°) for half an hour.

Meanwhile, make a thick Béchamel sauce with 2 heaped tablespoons of butter, $1\frac{1}{2}$ of flour and $\frac{3}{4}$–1 pint of milk. Add salt, pepper, a little cinnamon or nutmeg. Put a bay leaf into it and leave there while the sauce cools. When it is tepid remove the bay leaf and add 1 egg, beaten well with a fork.

Take the casserole out of the oven, pour the sauce carefully over and replace to cook for another hour of until the top is set and just browning.

Total cooking time is about $1\frac{1}{2}$ hours but, like many Greek dishes of its kind, this one can be left in a very low oven for many hours. It comes to no harm and possibly improves.

62. Grilling of Meat

Ulcer diets generally recommend grilling, as opposed to frying, as the method for cooking chops, steaks and other tender cuts of meat. The directions for doing so are simple enough:

1. The meat should always be removed from the refrigerator at least a couple of hours before eating.

2. Olive or other vegetable oil, not butter or lard, should be brushed over the meat—this is better done some time before cooking.

3. The grill should be pre-heated at its highest setting well before grilling begins.

4. The meat should first be browned on each side for 2–3 minutes, the grill then turned down. The whole cooking time will depend upon the thickness of the meat and may take from 10–25 minutes.

So much for the simple directions. For me, they don't always work. Grilling is too important a part of ulcer cookery for me to pass lightly over this point.

Meat under my grill, however long pre-heated, does not always brown as it should. The juices sometimes escape. The heat necessary to seal these in may easily cause some fat in the pan to burn. This upsets stomachs like mine.

I used to think that the fault was mine. But comparing results with other cooks I believe that the trouble is with the cookers. Many small domestic cookers simply don't provide the intense and steady heat necessary to produce the desired results.

If yours does, good luck to you. But if, like me, you have difficulty, then I suggest that baking is a better way of treating chops, for instance. It does not require the same undivided last-minute attention as grilling, nor involve the likelihood of burning fat.

63. Baked Chops

Veal, lamb, or in untroubled periods even the occasional pork chop can be cooked in an oiled shallow ovenproof pan, taking on average ½ hour in a well-heated oven. The chops can be flavoured with herbs, or with sliced onions—but the latter should not be served to the person with the ulcer.

64. Baked Lamb Cutlets

2 *cutlets per person* (or 1 *chump chop*)
cooking oil
butter
mint

Into a shallow oven dish put a little cooking oil. Brush this over the cutlets and bake them in a pre-heated oven at 400° for 35–40 minutes. Look at them after 20 minutes and lower heat if necessary.

Chop the leaves of mint finely and work into butter (about 1 teaspoonful per cutlet). When the cutlets are done, pour off all the fat from the pan and put a spoonful of mint butter on each. Serve as this begins to melt.

65. Navarin Printanier

A stew of lamb and spring vegetables, this is simpler than it sounds. It needs no attention during its long cooking except for the adding of the vegetables. It is a complete meal in itself.

2–3 *lb. shoulder of lamb*
4 *small onions*
a bunch of new carrots
1 *lb. new potatoes*
½ *lb. small turnips*
1½ *lb. new peas* (3 *lb. unshelled*)
rosemary
garlic
butter
salt

Buy a piece of shoulder of lamb of the right weight (a half shoulder, usually) unrolled. With a sharp knife remove the bone. Put the bone to boil with an onion, a carrot, a bay leaf and 3 peppercorns.

Cut the meat into 2-inch cubes, removing skin, gristle, anything that will not emerge soft from the cooking. Prepare all the vegetables: scrub the carrots and potatoes, peel the turnips (quarter them if they are at all big), shell the peas and slice the onions, having removed completely the outer sphere if it contains any hard, papery skin.

Choose a thick pan which will hold all the ingredients comfortably. Put first the onions, and then the squares of meat, into 3 tablespoons of butter. Do not fry, but let them take colour gently. Remove them, add 2 tablespoons of flour to the butter and mix into a smooth paste. Strain the stock made of the bone and vegetables and add about ½ pint of it slowly, while it is still hot, to the pan to make a light brown sauce. Return the meat and the onions to this, add salt, no pepper and a branch of rosemary and clove of garlic. Cook for an hour, either on the lowest heat or in a slow oven.

Add the potatoes, carrots and turnips. Continue to cook for 30–40 minutes, then add the peas. In 20–30 minutes taste the peas. If they are soft, serve. Remove the rosemary and garlic before you do. Total cooking time: about 2½ hours.

66. Skewered Lamb

This way of cooking cubes of meat threaded on skewers is not very troublesome. It enables you easily to provide only the lean, digestible flesh. This cooks quickly and satisfactorily under the ordinary grill.

It is therefore well worth mastering and doing often. Good recipes turn up under many names—kebabs, souvlakia, shashlik, and other words in the languages of the countries of the Middle East and Asia where they originate. I give only two, for lamb and liver, because kebabs of beef don't seem different enough from plain grilled steak to be worth making.

But by all means, if you like, follow other recipes. Don't, I suggest, thread on vegetables with the meat which will either, like tomatoes, fall off; or like onions, remain raw and cause upsets. Don't either include vinegar or lemon juice in any marinades for the meat, as in my experience they only harden it and make it taste sour.

leg or *shoulder of lamb*
($\frac{1}{4}$–$\frac{1}{2}$ lb. per person)
olive oil
bay leaves
lemon
rosemary, *if possible*

Ordinary butcher's skewers will do, but the longer flat-bladed ones you can buy now make the kebabs easier to turn over.

Leg of lamb is all lean, and expensive. Shoulder is cheaper, and more trouble. You must decide.

Either you or your butcher should cut the meat into 2-inch squares, free of all skin or gristle.

Thread the cubes on to the skewers, with a bay leaf every two or three pieces. Do one skewer for each person.

Lay the completed skewers in a shallow dish and pour over a little olive oil. Leave them for an hour or so and turn them over once.

Cook them under the hottest grill possible for 15 minutes, turning them once or twice and brushing over the remaining oil. Serve with slices of lemon.

If you can get fresh rosemary, put a branch or two in with the meat awaiting cooking and then lay them underneath as you grill.

67. Skewered Liver and Bacon

½ lb. liver (see below)
¼ lb. lean bacon
olive oil
fresh sage leaves, if available (bay leaves if not)

Cover the liver with boiling water. Leave for 5 minutes.

Remove and cut into 1½-inch squares. In the process, remove every single piece of pipe or skin, leaving only sound meat.

Divide the pieces into two piles (one for each person). Cut the bacon into roughly as many pieces as you have of liver, cutting away all rind, gristle and most fat. Divide the bacon equally between the two piles of liver.

Thread on to skewers about 6 inches long, in the order bacon, liver, sage leaf, and so on. If you use bay leaves, 1 or 2 per skewer is enough. Put completed skewers into a dish and pour over 3 tablespoons olive oil. Leave at least 15 minutes, and preferably longer. Put under a pre-heated grill turned on full. Brush liberally with olive oil during grilling. Grill for 2–3 minutes on each side to brown and seal in the juices. Grill about 5 minutes on each side and serve.

Only calf's or lamb's liver should be served to someone with an ulcer. It can, if you prefer, be simply grilled, in slices, in the same way described in the recipe. For the tenderest and mildest of liver you can forego the process of covering with boiling water.

Ox, sheep and pig's liver should play no part in the ulcer diet, though I suggest one use for the last in my Borderline Dishes.

68. Ham in White Sauce

Ham isn't ideal ulcer food. Older diets used to forbid it, but in real life a meal sometimes has to be prepared when ham, tinned or bought in slices, is much the best basis available.

I've never found it upsetting, simply served plain. But it is certainly both more appealing and more soothing heated up in a sauce. The way I suggest includes, I hope, nothing you would not ordinarily have in the house and nothing expensive.

½ *lb. cold cooked ham*	¾ *pint milk*
2 *tablespoons butter*	1 *small onion*
2 *tablespoons flour*	*seasonings*

Peel the onion and remove outer sphere. Chop finely. Melt the butter, soften the onion in it for 5 minutes, add the flour and cook for another 3 minutes. Add the heated milk slowly and put in any of the following seasonings you may have: bay leaf, juniper berries, mace, peppercorns. Cook on a very low heat or over boiling water for ½ hour, stirring occasionally. Put sauce through the Mouli, pour over the slices of ham in a shallow oven dish and heat in a low oven (310°) for 15 minutes.

69. Boiled Beef

2½–3 *lb. silverside* or *other beef for boiling*	10 *peppercorns*
1 *large onion*	4 *cloves*
2 *leeks, if available*	*parsley*
2 *large carrots*	1 *tablespoon salt*

Tell the butcher what you want the beef for so that he will roll and tie it securely.

Peel the vegetables, split and wash the leeks if you include them. Wash a small handful of parsley.

Three-quarters fill with water a pan big enough to hold everything and bring it to the boil. Put in the meat and, after the pan returns to the boil, skim the scum from the water for the next 5 minutes. Turn the heat down to the lowest reading and put in the other ingredients.

Continue to cook gently for 1½–2 hours, on top or in a low oven.

Serve the beef with steamed carrots and, if you like, creamed potatoes.

70. Meat Loaf

1 lb. minced steak
1 onion
6 tomatoes
½ pint breadcrumbs
2 eggs
1 rasher bacon diced small
1 dessertspoon soy sauce
butter
seasonings
parsley

Have the meat minced for you by the butcher, including no skin, fat or gristle.

Peel and chop the onion, chop 3 washed but unpeeled tomatoes. Simmer them together for 20 minutes in 2 tablespoons stock or water, with 4 peppercorns and a piece of mace. Put through the Mouli into a large bowl, add breadcrumbs, meat, bacon, the eggs beaten with a fork, the soy sauce, a handful of chopped parsley, 1 teaspoon salt. Mix thoroughly.

Before washing up the Mouli, put through 3 more chopped raw tomatoes to use later.

Line a 1-lb. loaf tin with oiled foil and put in the mixture. Put a bay leaf on top. Stand in a pan of water and bake at 350° for 1½–2 hours, until the top looks browned.

When the meat loaf is almost ready, heat up the 3 sieved tomatoes in 1 tablespoon butter with more chopped parsley. Decant the loaf the right way up on to a hot plate and pour the sauce over or serve it separately in a jug.

71. Hamburgers

¼ lb. minced lean beef per person
cooking oil

Have the butcher mince specially for you, or mince yourself, the beef, free of all fat or gristle. Shape each ¼ lb. into a flat cake. Just before cooking, brush with oil. Put under a pre-heated grill at its highest setting and brown on each side for 3–4 minutes. Turn down grill to its lowest setting and cook each side for another 3–4 minutes.

72. Braised Beef with Summer Vegetables

1 lb. braising steak in large pieces
2 bunches new carrots
1 onion
a few new turnips
stock
flour
butter
seasonings

Most good recipes for stewing cheap cuts of beef start by frying the meat and onions. This is an exception that works well. The meat I use is shoulder steak.

Cut up the onion and 6 of the carrots, scrubbed. In a thick pan with a lid make a bed of them, some herbs (thyme, marjoram, parsley), a teaspoon of salt, 6 peppercorns. Put the pieces of meat on this and pour over enough heated stock to come half-way up them. Put on the lid and cook very gently for 4 hours.

Remove the pieces of meat and keep them warm. Put stock, vegetables and herbs through the food mill. In another pan blend 1 tablespoon of flour into 1½ tablespoons of butter. When the flour has browned add slowly the stock mixture and stir until smooth. Put into this the remaining new carrots, scraped, and new turnips (about 1 to every 3 carrots), peeled and quartered. Put the pieces of meat over them and cook 45 minutes or so until the vegetables are soft. Scatter with chopped parsley and serve with good bread or toast.

73. Stewed Shin of Beef

Many cheap cuts of beef are all fat or gristle, but shin is leaner, so more useful. The recipe which introduced me to this cut is a good one to end the section. It is a celebration dish, only for a good period. Use bacon, not salt pork, less garlic or none, only a tablespoon of wine, with more stock. Most important, strain out herbs and onions from the sauce before serving.

For permission to print the recipe, from her *French Provincial Cooking*, published by Michael Joseph, I am grateful to Elizabeth David.

'Cut 4–6 oz. of fat bacon or salt pork into little cubes and put them, with a tablespoon of olive oil, into a heavy and fairly wide iron or earthenware pot; when the bacon fat runs add a large sliced onion. On top, arrange about 3 lb. of shin of beef, off the bone, skin and excess fat removed, and cut lengthways into thick pieces. Add a clove or two of garlic and a big bunch of parsley, thyme and bay leaf, all tied with a thread. Pour in a large glass (6–8 fl. oz.) of red wine, previously heated. Let it come to a fast boil and leave 3 or 4 minutes. Add an equal quantity of hot water, or stock should you chance to have it, and allow to boil again. Season with 2 teaspoons of salt.

'Cover the pot with paper or foil and a well-fitting lid. Transfer to a very slow oven, 290°F., and in about 3 hours it will be cooked. Or you can half-cook it one day and finish the process just as slowly the next, for . . . wine stews improve and mature with reheating. The sauce is to be neither thickened nor reduced; it is to be mopped up with plenty of bread, rice or potatoes. And if your oven is too small for your cooking-pot, then it can simmer extremely gently on top of the stove. There should be enough for six people.'

Borderline Dishes

74. Game
    Stewed pigeons
75. Shepherd's pie
76. Pork and gammon
    Boiled gammon
    Boiled joint of pork
77. Pot roast
78. Liver pâté

INTRODUCTION

I have warned in the main introduction, and I repeat here, the few dishes in this section are unconventional ones for a collection of this kind and are only to be used when the ulcer has been quiet for a long time. I then think that these will provide a better-judged foray into the slightly more colourful range of foods than might otherwise take place.

I have tested these particularly thoroughly, on myself, and on friends with ulcers.

74. Game

The older ulcer diets flatly ruled out all game. Few sufferers when feeling queasy would disagree with them. The strong flavour of wild things is altogether too much at such times.

But in a good period, some people at least may want a safe way of enjoying the gamey taste once in its season. I summarize my own experience:

Wild duck. Tried it, loved it, made extremely ill by it.

Pheasant: Delicious and safe when roasted but the tender birds necessary for this are expensive.

Hare: Jugged, too rich. (For this book I tried out many recipes for roasting saddle of hare. The recipes were fine but the hares varied a great deal, including some so tough they made me ill. I decided to leave out hare.)

Pigeons: These, which are the cheapest form of game I can buy, have never given me anything but pleasure. Accordingly, I follow with my recipe for them, which is only slightly varied from those given in many cookery books from Eliza Acton onwards.

Stewed Pigeons

2 *pigeons*
4 *oz. bacon*
4 *oz. mushrooms*
1 *large onion* or 3–4 *small ones*
butter
1 *tablespoon brandy*, *whisky* or *other spirit*
1 *cup stock* or *water*
seasonings

You need a covered oven dish that can be used on the top as well, large enough to hold the pigeons. Wash them in cold water, shake them dry and in this dish let them take colour lightly in one tablespoon of butter. Turn them over carefully and don't let the butter burn.

Meanwhile, in a thick frying-pan, the washed whole mushrooms and the onions should also be very lightly cooked in 2 tablespoons of butter.

(Whether you use 1 big onion, peeled and sliced, or the much nicer, but scarcer small ones, do not serve them, only pigeon and mushrooms, to the ulcer sufferer.)

Into the pan with the pigeons pour a tablespoon of brandy, whisky, or almost any spirit you may have. It is not essential but it seems to help to soften the pigeons in cooking. Let it bubble for a couple of minutes.

Add the now lightly cooked onions and mushrooms, 1 cup of hot stock or water, a little salt and 6 peppercorns. Cook the bacon for about 2 minutes on each side in the mushroom-and-onion pan and spread the pieces neatly over the pigeons. These should sit side by side, breast up in their pan.

Cover, cook in a low oven, 325°, for 2 hours.

Many recipes give shorter cooking times but the birds I buy, which are shot locally, take all of 2 hours. Longer cooking, at a slightly lower temperature, does them no harm.

Eliza Acton suggests stuffing the birds with more small mushrooms, lightly cooked in butter.

75. Shepherd's Pie

1 lb. beef minced for you
1½ lb. potatoes
1 medium-sized onion
¼ lb. mushrooms
3 tablespoons breadcrumbs
1 tablespoon soy sauce
butter
seasonings

The meat must not be butcher's mince, but rump or other lean beef minced specially for you (or by you) and containing no fat or gristle. The breadcrumbs too should not be the bought kind, but made by you, of toasted bread, grated, crushed or put into the blender.

Peel the potatoes and the onion and boil them together in just enough water to cover, with 6 peppercorns, 1 teaspoon salt, and a bay leaf. When tender, put through the Mouli, adding 1 tablespoon butter and just a little of their cooking water to make a creamy purée.

Put the butter into a large frying-pan. *Do not proceed to fry.* On the lowest heat your cooker produces, just melt the butter. The moment it melts put in the meat, and turn it about for 3–5 minutes. Add the whole washed mushrooms, and mix them lightly with the meat for another 3–5 minutes. Add breadcrumbs, soy sauce, and a sprinkling of nutmeg. Mix all lightly together and remove from heat.

Put the meat mixture into a buttered pie dish, pour over the purée of potatoes and onions and make criss-crosses on top with a fork. Bake at 425° for 45 minutes, or until the top just browns.

76. Pork and Gammon

These meats were once totally banned from the ulcer diet and they are still not generally recommended. If in doubt you should ask your doctor's advice and follow it.

For those on a looser rein, I suggest that if you have them

at all you do not roast but boil them. I do not say that families will all think this way of cooking as good as roasting: most children will miss pork crackling, and the browned skin of roast gammon. But both of these, it can be definitely said, will upset any ulcer. And most families will prefer these quite pleasant ways of serving pork or gammon to the alternative of never eating them at all.

Boiled Gammon

The piece of gammon should be very firmly and thoroughly tied into shape. Soak it in cold water for 2 or 3 hours, and pour this away. Put the meat into a large pan with 6 peppercorns, 3 cloves, a bay leaf, an onion, and a carrot. Bring it gradually to a bare boil, and keep it there, only just simmering. Skim off scum for 5 minutes with a slotted spoon. Continue to cook very slowly for 40 minutes per pound. Gammon cooked this way is good hot or cold. Either way, it should be very thinly sliced.

Boiled joint of Pork

The piece of pork, a good lean roasting cut, should be boned and firmly tied. In a big thick pan put 2 tablespoons of cooking oil, and in this over a medium heat turn the pork about to brown it evenly. Take the pan off the burner, take out the pork and pour away every drop of the oil, wiping the pan with a paper towel. Replace the joint, put the pan back on a lowered heat and instantly pour in enough boiling water to come a third of the way up the meat. When it boils, turn the heat down as low as it will go. Add 2 teaspoons of salt, 6 peppercorns, thyme, sage, an onion, a carrot.

Cook as slowly as you can. A joint weighing about 2½ lb. will take 1½–2 hours to cook. This, too, is good eaten hot or cold. The strained liquid, chilled and with the fat skimmed off, is a beautifully flavoured stock to use, for instance, to make a thick vegetable soup.

77. Pot Roast

2½–3 lb. rolled beef (*see below*)
1 rasher bacon
1 large onion
2 tomatoes
2 carrots
1 stick celery
½ lb. small mushrooms
¼ pint stock or *water*
herbs
seasonings

This dish represents the limit I would risk of departure from the old strict ulcer diets. I have suffered no ill-effects from it but I would not eat it in any but a long untroubled period. If in doubt, serve instead the boiled beef on p. 103.

The meat can be any cut the butcher normally sells for pot roasting, but it must be prepared without the roll of fat in which such cuts are normally encased. It should be well-tied into a roll.

Cut the bacon into small squares and put into a frying pan on a low heat. When the fat runs add the sliced onion and cook very gently until it has softened. Lift with a slotted spoon into a thick casserole of cast iron or earthenware. Put the meat into the frying pan and brown it very lightly for 5–10 minutes. Lift it into the casserole. Add the sliced carrots, peeled and chopped tomatoes and celery cut into short lengths. Pour over ¼ pint heated stock or water, bring to the boil, immediately turn down and add 1 bay leaf, 4 peppercorns, mace and dried or fresh thyme. Cook very slowly on top, or in a low oven (275°), for 3–4 hours. Turn the meat over once or twice.

An hour before serving, remove from the vegetables all the fat you can with a bulb baster, put them through the Mouli and return them to the meat pan with the washed whole mushrooms to cook for the last hour. Serve with noodles.

78. Liver Pâté

1½ lb. pig's liver
4 oz. bacon
1 onion
4 heaped tablespoons butter
2 juniper berries and other seasonings

Wash the liver well and trim off all fat or membrane. Cover it with boiling water, leave for 5 minutes and then drain. Peel and slice the onion, removing all papery or tough outside pieces. Stew gently in the butter in a thick-bottomed saucepan over the lowest heat for 5–10 minutes, until soft. Stir the slices about so that they cook evenly and on no account turn up the heat. Put through the finest blade of the mincer the liver, all but two rashers of bacon, and the onions. Turn up the mincer to get every drop of the butter in which the onion stewed, and don't leave any behind in the pan. Two juniper berries, minced with the liver, make a great difference to the flavour of the dish. Add a little grated nutmeg, a little grated pepper and a teaspoon of salt. If you have it, a teaspoon of brandy can be added; and if it will be popular in your house, a crushed clove of garlic. I make this frequently without either.

Mix the ingredients well together. Your fingers make the best job of this. Put the mixture into a 2-pint oven-proof dish, which can be either the French cast iron rectangular one made for the purpose, or a soufflé dish, preferably a thick one; or simply a loaf tin. Put a bay leaf on top and surround this by the two rashers of bacon cut into thin strips.

Stand the dish in a baking-tin of water and cook it uncovered in a low oven, 310°, for 1½ hours. The pâté should by then be standing free of the sides of the dish. Let it cool, then put a plate or something else flat which fits into the dish with a weight of some kind on it and leave overnight. You can turn the pâté out on to a dish before serving, with French bread or toast. It will keep for a week in the refrigerator.

The pâté makes a good summer lunch, followed by some suitable salad; or a pleasant supper, preceded by eggs of some kind. It sounds an odd dish for an ulcer diet, but I advance it with confidence, having served it many times to ulcerated as well as more fortunate friends. To my surprise it proves popular with children.

Vegetables

79. Bouquet of steamed vegetables
80. Steamed carrots
81. Steamed leeks
82. Purées of root vegetables
    - parsnips
    - swedes
    - young turnips
    - beetroot
    - carrots
    - celeriac and potatoes
83. Creamed potatoes
84. Potatoes in casserole
85. Cucumbers
    - in white sauce
    - in butter with dill
    - in cream
86. Broad beans
    - Old broad beans
    - Broad bean purée
87. Fresh green peas
88. Baby beetroot
    - boiled, with butter and herbs
    - baked, with cream
89. Swiss chard
90. Courgettes
    - with herbs
    - baked with tomatoes
91. Jerusalem artichokes
92. Cauliflower with lemon butter

Since doubts have been raised about leaf vegetables, I have excluded them. I myself have had troubles traceable directly to tinned spinach, to sorrel, to cabbage and to sprouts, so I avoid these. Purée of fresh spinach is included in some works on ulcer cookery, so obviously need not be denied to anyone fond of and unharmed by it.

Any part of a vegetable which will not cook tender will cause trouble and common sense will tell you what these are: skins of old broad beans, or of stringy runner beans, or the hard outer stalks of celery. In general, young and tender vegetables are much better for those with ulcers. In the winter, when these are scarce, purées of root vegetables take over. Some may think this programme a deprivation but I am not one of them.

79. Bouquet of Steamed Vegetables

I put this way of cooking first because it so simplifies the whole procedure of catering for an ulcer.

To steam vegetables satisfactorily, you need a steamer of some kind. The little French gadget that sits in an ordinary saucepan is cheap and convenient. There are also special saucepans with a top piece like a double boiler with holes in it. You can steam in an ordinary colander, if you have a saucepan big enough to take it. But this is clumsy and only worth doing once to find out if you really like the method.

For me, it has transformed vegetable cookery. Vegetables steamed together keep their individual flavours: bouquet is not too fancy a word for the effect. They go well with simply cooked meat or fish. They are also delicious with boiled beef or *poule au pot*, or any other dish which produces a flavour-some liquid.

Vegetables

What vegetables you use, and in what proportions, is up to you. So you can leave out what you or your children dislike, or put in more of what they do like. You can make the bouquet of what you find on sale. You can use up what you have left in the larder, since quantities are not critical.

Neither is timing. The process is slower than others so that if the vegetables cook longer than you intended, they will not be ruined.

Here is a typical, straightforward bouquet:

2 *potatoes*
4 *carrots*
1 *small onion*
1 *stick of celery*
parsley

Peel the vegetables and cut them into pieces roughly the same size. Take particular care over the onion, rejecting all tough outer pieces. Cut the tender centre into thin, even slices. Fill the saucepan to just below the steamer with water and when it is boiling put in the carrots, celery and onion. Five minutes later put in the potatoes. Scatter over $\frac{1}{2}$ teaspoon of salt and steam on a low heat for 25 minutes. Taste. If the vegetables are tender, scatter chopped parsley over them and cook another 2 or 3 minutes. If not, wait 5 minutes, taste again. When the vegetables are cooked, add the parsley.

So much for the basic method. But the joy—and the convenience—is in the variations:

1. I have used leeks, peas, cucumber, young white turnips, celeriac in bouquets. (Marrows, young or old, are not good in them and green beans do not respond well to steaming at all.)

About 3 vegetables seems enough to me and more than 4 to be over-complicated.

2. More delicate herbs, like chervil or tarragon or dill, can be used and reveal their taste more in this than in almost any other way.

3. You will vary the time of cooking to suit your and your family's preferences. Undercooked vegetables are not good for ulcerated stomachs, overcooked ones are not pleasant for others. Steaming broadens the area of choice for you. You will, obviously, put in hard vegetables like carrots, turnips and celery a little before the others and you will cook the bouquet longer if the steamer is full. Only small onions should ever be used and of these only the tender parts near the centre.

4. By varying the vegetables and herbs you use, you can, in a busy time, serve these bouquets night after night without, I think, boring those for whom you cook. I think that, in real life, there is seldom time anyway to prepare the elaborate vegetable dishes I read of in cookery books; and ulcer cookery is more time-consuming than most. For those who haven't come across it, this way of doing vegetables is a genuine discovery.

Steaming is, too, the best way of cooking some vegetables individually. Here are two examples:

80. Steamed Carrots

Many ulcer sufferers, including me, find plain boiled carrots, although safe, slightly sickening. Stewing in their own juice over-sweetens them, in the case of tinned carrots disgustingly so.

This way is better: peel the carrots or scrape them, chop the big ones in two and cut them into matchsticks. Steam them 15–20 minutes with $\frac{1}{2}$ teaspoon of salt on top. About 5 minutes before serving scatter chopped parsley and squeeze some lemon juice over them. Serve butter with them.

New carrots, scraped and left whole, are excellent cooked this way.

81. Steamed Leeks

A sure way to make leeks both palatable and digestible is this one: cut the root end well away and every bit of green stem from the other. Split them, discard any outer pieces that look at all tough or stringy, wash them well. Place them neatly side by side in the steamer, salt and steam 10–15 minutes. Taste to be sure they are tender. Squeeze a little lemon juice over them and serve with butter.

If you have time, instead of butter and lemon juice, make the hot tomato and lemon sauce described for baked fish on p. 76 and pour over the leeks at the last minute.

82. Purées of Root Vegetables

Sieved vegetables used to play a great part in the old strict gastric diets, and crudely mashed vegetables in the school meals of our childhoods. These unappetizing dishes have left behind a strong prejudice, both among the ulcerated and those of healthy stomach, against this way of cooking.

Yet carefully-made and well-seasoned vegetable purées are served in the world's best restaurants, and no wonder. They look appealing, they taste good in themselves and are unequalled for bringing out the flavour of simply grilled or roast meats. And, since any hard fibrous matter has been strained out or chopped finely, these purées are easy on the stomach, as their presence on the old diet sheets suggests.

They aren't much trouble to prepare, with the right equipment.

Vegetable sieves are tedious to use, and to wash up. The French Moulin-Légumes, more often simply called the Mouli, is a far better device and comparatively cheap.

I see no reason for those who don't have one already, and aren't rich, to rush to buy an expensive electric blender in order to cater for an ulcer. Useful as these machines are, they do produce a texture of which people can quickly tire, especially ulcer sufferers who have eaten so much baby food in their time. The Mouli is a little more work, but not much, and I myself prefer the fluffier, less even, more French appearance of its purées.

For the recipes that follow you can, unless otherwise indicated, use either the Mouli, a blender, or should you prefer, a sieve.

The mixtures should be neither too wet nor too dry. Although I have arrived most painstakingly at the proportions I suggest, vegetables do vary in water content, so add liquids gradually and stop when the mixture is still stiff. The purée should stand up on the plate like a successful soufflé, with no liquid leaking out of it.

When an ulcer flares up, a meal of poached or baked eggs with a vegetable purée will help to calm it. You can make these purées of things other than the root crops I suggest here (there is a recipe for old broad beans on p. 126). But I think it is a pity to reduce to pulp a tender summer vegetable. To me, purées are wintry dishes, warming, filling —and quite sufficient in themselves without other vegetables.

Purée of Parsnips

2 lb. parsnips
2 oz. butter
2 dessertspoons cream
2 tablespoons stale white breadcrumbs
1 dessertspoon chopped parsley
salt

If you're hard pressed for time you can just boil parsnips tender, peel them, put them through the Mouli or into the blender, add butter, salt and reheat. The result is tolerable but this recipe is a more persuasive way to serve them.

Scrub the whole parsnips, cut off the stem ends and steam them 30 minutes. With a table knife strip off the skins, split the parsnips lengthways and remove what you can of the woody centres. Put them through the Mouli, add the butter, the cream, the parsley, 1 teaspoon salt and beat with a wooden spoon (or do this all in the blender). Spread in a soufflé dish, cover with the breadcrumbs and a few more dots of butter and re-heat in an oven set at 400°.

Two tablespoons of grated mild Cheddar can be added to the purée before re-heating to make it more substantial and nourishing.

Eggs cooked in ramekins (p. 44) go well with this purée and together they make a good lunch.

Purée of Swedes

1 *swede weighing* 1–1½ *lb.*
2 *tablespoons meat stock* or *consommé*
2 *oz. butter*
2 *tablespoons brown breadcrumbs*
1 *teaspoon lemon juice*
seasonings

Peel the swedes, cut them into cubes and boil them until soft —only 10–15 minutes—in salted water with 3 peppercorns and a bay leaf. Put through the Mouli, add butter, lemon juice, and the stock. This should be quite concentrated, either some you've reduced by boiling or the jelly (free of fat) saved from a roast; or good tinned consommé. Beat with a wooden spoon, spread in a soufflé dish with the breadcrumbs on top, heat through in the oven set at 400°.

This is worth trying once on those who are suspicious of swedes.

Purée of Young Turnips

Turnips cooked this way are pleasant and harmless to eat. But they still taste of turnips, which many people, especially children, loathe. As the dish is quite a lot of trouble be sure of your audience before you bother.

2 lb. young white turnips
2 oz. butter
2 tablespoons cream

Boil the peeled, quartered turnips fast in just enough water to cover them, with salt and 3 peppercorns. Test with a skewer after 10 minutes, and cook until tender. Put them through a Mouli (not into a blender). What comes through will be fairly liquid. Reduce this by boiling, stirring to stop it from sticking. When most of the liquid has gone, take the pan off the burner, add the butter, the cream and beat with a wooden spoon. Heat up again, stirring as you do, and serve.

Purée of Beetroot

1 lb. cooked beetroot
2 tablespoons chicken stock
1 tablespoon butter
2 teaspoons lemon juice
salt

This is an excellent winter dish, using cold beetroot from a decent greengrocer who will have cooked it properly.

Peel it, remove any imperfections, dice it roughly. Heat it up in the stock. Put it through the Mouli or into the blender; if the latter, let the blender run until all lumps are gone. Add the butter, the lemon juice and enough salt, which may be 2 teaspoons. Reheat on top or in the oven and serve with steak or any grilled meat.

Purée of Carrots

1 lb. carrots
1 small tomato or
juice of half a lemon
2 tablespoons butter
2 tablespoons cream
salt
herbs

When carrots are getting old and tough, this is a good way to treat them. Scrub them, cut off stem end, steam them

½ hour or until tender. With a table knife strip off the skins.

Put them through the Mouli or into the blender and add the cream, butter and 1 teaspoon of salt. If you are using the blender, dip the tomato into boiling water and skin it before adding; for the Mouli it can simply be washed, chopped and put through with the carrots. Use either tomato or lemon juice but not both.

When the purée is smoothly mixed, heat it up either on top or in a soufflé dish in the oven. Just before serving, add a bare teaspoon of chopped parsley, tarragon, chervil, or the best you can get.

Purée of Celeriac and Potato

Celeriac, when it turns up, is well worth including in the ulcer diet. On its own, even in a purée, it has too strong a flavour. But a mixture, half and half, with potatoes, makes perhaps the best purée of them all. Boil the peeled and sliced celeriac separately and then simply make a purée of it and the potatoes together, according to your usual method for creamed potatoes, or mine, which follows.

83. Creamed Potatoes

potatoes	*butter*
milk	*salt*

Cookery experts, and my friends, hold vehement opinions about this dish. My own is mild, and briefly stated. It is a good dish for ulcer sufferers and should be given to them often. If it takes too much trouble, many pans, whisks and such, it won't be.

Therefore, boil the potatoes in not too much water. Put them through the Mouli. Add butter, about 2 tablespoons per pound of potatoes. Heat the milk, and add enough to produce the consistency you like. Salt to suit yourself. Leave pepper to be added at the table. Reheat on a low burner, keep warm in a low oven or over hot water. Add a little finely chopped parsley before serving.

84. Potatoes in Casserole

Cookery books often contain good recipes for doing potatoes slowly in the oven. The results are almost always extremely soothing. The dish can be cooked while you have the oven on for something else, and is particularly useful if you are going to do something like grilling meat, which will take all your attention at the last minute.

This is only one of many such dishes that I can recommend. It combines so well the flavours of three vegetables that there is no point in serving any other with it.

It is adapted from Ambrose Heath, *Good Potato Dishes.*

2 *lb. potatoes*	3 *tablespoons butter*
1 *small onion*	1 *tablespoon flour*
2 *large* or 4 *small tomatoes*	¼ *pint taken from top of milk*

Chop the washed tomatoes into big pieces and press them raw through the Mouli. In the butter soften the finely chopped onion. Add flour and cook together for 3 minutes. Add the tomato purée and the milk and cook for another 3 minutes. Put this sauce through the Mouli.

Have the potatoes peeled and thinly sliced. Put them into the pan, turn them over until the sauce is distributed through them, put the whole lot into an earthenware casserole and bake at 375° for 1½ hours.

85. Cucumbers

Raw cucumbers will upset an ulcer. More puzzling to me is the report of many ulcer specialists that their patients find cooked cucumbers troublesome, too. I suspect that in these cases the cucumbers were improperly treated; that is, not drained of their acid juices before cooking. If you have doubts, do not introduce cucumbers into the diet. I have none, after many years of eating them cooked as I describe below.

Cucumbers in White Sauce

1 *large cucumber* or 2 *small ones*
1 *tablespoon butter*
1 *tablespoon flour*
$\frac{1}{2}$ *pint milk*
salt

Peel the cucumber and cut into quarters lengthwise. If it is large, with tough seeds, remove them. Cut the cucumber into thin strips about 2 inches long. Put these into a colander, salt them well and leave them for an hour. Rinse them in cold water and dry in a cloth.

In the top of the double boiler melt the butter directly over a low flame. Put in the cucumber and cook *extremely gently* for 5 minutes. Add the flour and mix together lightly. Gradually add the warmed milk and a little salt. Cook over boiling water for 15 minutes and serve.

Cucumbers in Butter with Dill

Prepare the cucumbers as above. When they are rinsed and dried cook them, again in a double saucepan, this time in 2 tablespoons butter. Add 1 tablespoon chopped dill and cook over boiling water for 15 minutes.

Cucumbers in Cream

Proceed as in the previous two recipes, but when the cucumbers have been cooked for 5 minutes in 1 tablespoon butter, remove from the heat and add 2 tablespoons double cream. Stir gently together and leave over boiling water for 25–30 minutes.

86. Broad Beans

When these beans are very young and tender they need only be boiled for 10 minutes or steamed for 12–15, and served with butter. (If you can be bothered, there are good recipes in many books for putting them into cream, yoghourt, or egg and lemon sauces.)

When broad beans are old they should not be served at all unless you can be bothered to take some time and trouble with them: to remove their tough skins, or to make a purée.

Old Broad Beans, Skinned

Put them, shelled, into fast-boiling water and keep it boiling hard for 3 minutes only. Drain them in a colander, run cold water over them and gently pull off the skins.

If ancient, the skinned beans will need up to another 10 minutes simmering in the smallest possible amount of water before adding a little butter, or cream and salt. If reasonably tender they can simply be heated up in the butter or cream slowly, for 5–10 minutes.

Taking off the skins is tedious and can't be hurried. I think the result is worth the effort.

Broad Bean Purée

1 *lb. old broad beans, in their pods*
1 *large potato* or 2 *small*
1 *leek* or 1 *onion*
milk
butter
salt

Recipes exist for purées of young beans but it seems pointless in an ulcer diet to put perfectly acceptable tender vegetables through the food mill. I suggest this method be reserved for the tough old beans which demand it.

Wash them, cut off the stem ends and cut the beans into 2-inch lengths. Put them like this, pods and all, into only

1 inch of boiling salted water with 2 peppercorns. About 15 minutes later add the quartered potato and either the onion, quartered, or the leek, cut in half lengthways and well washed.

Cook slowly another ½ hour and put through the Mouli. While you're doing this, what little liquid is left in the pan can be reduced by boiling and can then be added to the purée. Taste and add more salt if necessary. Add 1 tablespoon butter and enough heated milk to produce a creamy, but not too liquid, texture.

This is almost too filling as a vegetable with meat. It makes a good main dish if served with poached eggs on it. The eggs can be baked in the purée instead (see Baked Egg Dishes, p. 46). Grilled lean bacon can be serve on it, too, or both eggs and bacon.

87. Fresh Green Peas

The traditional English way to cook these, with a sprig of mint, a little sugar and salt, is the best one I know for people with ulcers. I prefer it anyway to the French and other recipes involving lettuce, onions, shallots, bacon or ham.

Reputable cookery experts disagree sharply about how long, and at what heat, to cook fresh peas. In my experience a fast boil will burst them, and just simmering, or better still, steaming, are the best ways. They take 10–20 minutes and you can only know when they are done by tasting one.

Sometimes they remain hard as little stones, however you cook them. This I now believe is the fault of the peas, which are probably the sold-off remains of a crop raised for canning or freezing. If this happens to you the only course open is to continue cooking them for 30–45 minutes, put them through the food mill, add butter or cream. They make a pleasant purée, admittedly a disappointment if you've paid a lot for them, but better than upsetting an ulcer.

88. Baby Beetroot

Some greengrocers in England now sell small uncooked beetroot. Others will get them for you if you ask. In a diet short of good fresh vegetables, they are welcome: pleasant to eat, undemanding to the cook and to the stomach.

In the two recipes that follow the cooking methods are interchangeable: you can bake them if you happen to have the oven on, boil them if not, and afterwards treat them in any of the ways suggested.

Beetroot, Boiled, with Butter and Herbs

Don't peel the beetroot. Cut off root end and stem, scrub, half cover in salted water, bring to the boil and keep them steadily there for 1–1½ hours. Test with a skewer to be sure they're soft right through.

Run cold water over them in a colander, rub off the skins with your fingers. Unless they are really tiny, slice or quarter them. Heat them up in a thick pan with, first, a generous squeeze of fresh lemon juice and then about a tablespoon of butter. Scatter chopped fresh herbs over them before serving: parsley, tarragon, chives or such of these as you can get.

Beetroot, Baked, with Cream

Instead of boiling, bake the beetroot (not peeled, but trimmed and scrubbed) in an open dish or on a baking-sheet. They will take 2–3 hours, depending on how hot the oven is. Test them for softness with a skewer and remove the skins.

If you have sour cream, pour 2 tablespoons over the beetroot and heat them up in it. If the cream is fresh, not sour, then give the beetroot a squeeze of lemon juice first, heat the cream just to the boil and pour it over them. The same mixture of fresh herbs mentioned in the previous recipe can also be added to the cream just before serving.

89. Swiss Chard (or Seakale Beet)

I don't apologize for including this uncommon vegetable. I have seen it in greengrocers, I have found it the easiest of vegetables to grow and I read that it is 'by no means a rare vegetable in our gardens'.*

The leaves can be cooked like spinach and given to the rest of the family when the ulcer sufferer is out.

For the whole family, ulcer sufferer included, the stems are, I think, delicious and underrated by cookery writers.

They can be simply washed, trimmed and put into a casserole with 2 tablespoons of water, 1 of butter, salt and 2 or 3 peppercorns. At 325° they will be done in 1–1¼ hours.

Alternatively, you can take them out after an hour and pour over them a thick cheese sauce, into which you stir what liquid remains in the casserole (minus the peppercorns). Put the dish back in the oven, uncovered, for 15–20 minutes.

Fillets of cod or other white fish can be baked in the cheese sauce to make a main dish.

90. Courgettes

The ulcer diet, a little short on good vegetables, should definitely include one lot of courgettes, or young marrows, when they are in season. (They are, by the way, exceptionally easy to grow, even for the least experienced gardener.)

Their flavour is pleasant but faint, and better when combined with other tastes. Frying in oil or butter, which most cookery books recommend, is no use for this one. I have suggested a simple way of serving them with herbs and a more complicated one with tomatoes. A recipe for stuffing them appears on p. 56 for cooking with minced meat on p. 96, and for serving cold on p. 137.

* John Organ, *Rare Vegetables* (Faber and Faber, 1960), whose advice for cooking I have adapted in my recipes.

Courgettes with Herbs

Wash the courgettes and peel them along their ridges, leaving a few stripes of skin. Slice them about ½ inch thick, put them into a colander, salt them well and leave for an hour or so while their bitter juices ooze out.

Wash them in cold water and then boil in salted water. Very small ones will need only 10 minutes but bigger ones 15. Drain thoroughly.

Meanwhile, chop finely the best selection of fresh herbs you can get together: parsley, chives, tarragon. Put these into a thick pan with butter and let the butter melt and heat through, but not burn. Put in the pieces of courgette and turn them about carefully in the butter, just to coat, not to cook them.

Use the butter generously, 2 tablespoons to a pound of courgettes. You can use good olive oil instead, or cream, which is particularly delicious.

Courgettes baked with Tomatoes

2 lb. courgettes
1 lb. tomatoes
parsley
garlic (if you like)
1 cup of breadcrumbs
3 tablespoons olive oil
seasonings

Prepare the courgettes as in the previous recipe but slice them more thinly—¼ inch.

While their bitter juices are draining off in the colander, wash the tomatoes and quarter them. Put 1 tablespoon of olive oil into a thick frying pan and in this stew the tomatoes extremely gently for 10 minutes. If you are going to use garlic, put a chopped clove into the tomatoes as they cook. Then put them through the finest sieve of the Mouli. Do not bother to wash the frying pan yet.

Chop the parsley—a good handful—and mix it with the breadcrumbs.

In the same frying-pan put 1 more tablespoon of olive oil and heat it up. *Remove it from the fire* and carefully put in the pieces of courgette, first drying each one with a tea towel. They will not fry, or cook at all, but just be turned over to coat each side with the hot oil.

As each piece is done, put into a flat oven dish and continue, adding more oil and heating it up as necessary. The courgettes should nearly fill the dish. Then pour over the tomato purée and make an even layer of the breadcrumbs and parsley. Add salt and a little pepper.

Bake in a hot oven, 425°. They will take between 1 and 1½ hours. Look at them after the hour and serve them when the moisture has cooked away and the crumbs lightly browned.

This sounds like a lot of bother, and it is. You won't want to do it more than once a year and the diet shouldn't include it any oftener, for it is not the lightest of dishes. But it is one of the best for introducing a little Mediterranean colour into the diet, in high summer, when ulcers are often quiet.

91. Jerusalem Artichokes

The distinctive flavour of this vegetable adds interest to the ulcer diet in winter. Most greengrocers now sell a recently developed form which is much easier to prepare.

Scrub the artichokes with a brush, boil them in very little salted water or steam them 10–20 minutes. Don't overcook them—use a skewer to tell when they are soft. Remove the skins with a dull table knife. Reheat carefully and serve with butter or in a well-flavoured white sauce.

92. Cauliflower with Lemon Butter

'Allow 1 medium-sized cauliflower for 4 people. Cut off stem and leaves and separate into 5 or 6 clusters of flowerets.

(This breaking into several pieces is optional, of course; it does not present so handsome a dish as the whole cauliflower, but it reduces the cooking time considerably and thereby improves the flavour and preserves the whiteness.) Wash thoroughly and leave immersed in cold water 10 minutes. Throw into rapidly boiling water and cook until the stem part is just tender. Drain thoroughly and place in a hot serving-dish. Melt 4 tablespoons of butter over hot water, add 2 teaspoons of boiled lemon juice and dribble over the cauliflower. Sprinkle lightly with salt if necessary.'

This simple recipe I quote, with permission which I gratefully acknowledge, from *Good Food for Bad Stomachs*, by Sara M. Jordan and Sheila Hibben, published in New York by Doubleday and Company, Inc. It is the best and safest way I've ever found to serve cauliflower. I melt the butter on a low burner with an asbestos mat; what is important is that it should only be warmed through and come nowhere near sizzling.

Salads and Cold Food

93. Vegetables for salads
94. Meat for cold meals
95. Cold pigeon fillets with cherries
96. Cold beetroot
97. Celeriac salad
98. Salad of cold courgettes
99. Rice salad
100. Mushroom salad
101. Tomatoes in cream
102. Avocado pears
103. Salad of new potatoes
104. Cauliflower salad
105. A plate of young vegetables
106. Cold egg and lemon sauce
107. Boiled salad dressing
108. Mayonnaise

INTRODUCTION

The time of year when salads appear in England is dangerous for those with ulcers. This turn of the seasons, no one knows quite why, often reawakens an ulcer that has been quiet all winter. At such times, unfortunately, many people who cook, not wanting to waste hours of sunshine in a hot kitchen, turn to the sorts of salads and cold food which need no preparation: raw cucumber, watercress, radishes, tomatoes eaten skin and all, served with cold pork pies, or sausage rolls.

Each of these will quite certainly exacerbate an already tender stomach. Salads that suit an ulcer are not so effort-free, though goodness knows they are little enough trouble. I have given only a few as examples. Almost any vegetable in the previous section, cooked neither too little nor too much, is good served cold with a dressing.

Many friends with ulcers like and have no trouble with lettuce. It upsets me. Here, personal experience must dictate your choice. If eaten, it should be in the form of the tender inner leaves, dressed with oil and lemon juice, not vinegar.

There is no obvious reason why sandwiches should cause trouble yet most of us find that a meal of them is unwise. Once in a way, at a good period, you may want to risk it. A sandwich lunch every day is not a good idea.

Similarly, a picnic for the likes of us is better not dominated by bread, but including some cold meat, an acceptable salad of some kind, cheese or a cold sweet dish. This, too, is more trouble than pitching raw fruit and vegetables into a basket; but it certainly is not less pleasant to eat, whether you have an ulcer or not.

93. Vegetables for Salads

Here I summarize my suggestions. This list excludes some

good but unclassifiable cold foods to be found in the recipes themselves.

Vegetables recommended for use in salads:

- lettuce (as explained)
- avocados
- cooked beetroot
- cooked cauliflower
- cooked celeriac
- cooked courgettes
- cooked potatoes
- other cooked vegetables (see recipes)
- tomatoes (see recipe)

Vegetables not recommended for use in salads:

- grated raw vegetables of any kind
- cabbage
- celery
- green peppers
- radishes
- spring onions
- whole unpeeled tomatoes
- watercress

94. Meat for Cold Meals

Many of the recipes in other sections produce leftovers of meat which can be the centre of a cold meal:

Boiled or Baked Chicken (pp. 82–83)
Boiled Beef (p. 103)
Meat Loaf (p. 104)
Duck, Goose and Turkey (pp. 87–89)
Roast Veal (p. 89)
Boiled Pork (p. 110)
Boiled Gammon (p. 110)

The Liver Pâté (p. 113) is ideal for a cold meal, of course. The fish section contains a recipe for a codling served cold (p. 77). Many other large fish are good cold. They can be poached, or baked in foil, and can be served with any of the cold sauces suggested in this section.

If the meat, or other main course, is scarce, a few hard-boiled eggs help to fill it out. Some people find these hard to digest but I feel sure this is only because the eggs have been cooked until they are like rocks. Put into cold water, brought to the boil and cooked for 7–8 minutes, they seem to me perfectly all right.

95. Cold Pigeon Fillets with Cherries

Put the pigeons breast down in a pan with a lid, cover them in water and add salt, peppercorns, bay leaf, and such dried or fresh herbs as you have. Cover and cook extremely slowly on top or in an oven set at 300° for 2–3 hours, testing with a skewer to be sure they are tender. Let them cool in their own liquid.

Before serving, take off the fillets from either side of the breast with a dull table knife and remove the skin. Arrange them in a shallow dish and pour over and around them a compôte of cherries, made as described on p. 151.

96. Cold Beetroot

Cut small beetroot, boiled or baked (p. 128) and peeled, into matchsticks and put warm into a dressing of oil, lemon juice, salt. Leave for several hours or overnight and scatter with chopped parsley. Much better than bought ready-cooked beetroot, for which see the purée recommended on p. 122.

97. Celeriac Salad

Celeriac, peeled, cut into matchsticks, put into cold salted water, brought to the boil, kept there 3–5 minutes, drained in a colander, mixed with thin mayonnaise ($\frac{1}{2}$ cup to 1 celeriac root), scattered with finely chopped parsley, cooled: this, perhaps surprisingly, is one of the safest of salads.

It is best eaten at the start of a meal, I think. The cooking water is valuable for soups.

98. Salad of Cold Courgettes

Only very small courgettes are good cold, I think: not more than 4 inches long. Wash them, cut off the ends, boil them in salted water for 10 minutes. Put them in a colander to drain for ½ hour or so, then into a dressing of olive oil, lemon juice, salt and a little pepper. Turn them about and spoon the dressing over them a couple of times, and again just before serving.

99. Rice Salad

Boil a cup of Italian rice until it is just cooked, rinse it in hot water and while it is still warm mix into it a dressing of 2 tablespoons olive oil, the juice of ½ lemon and salt. Grate and mix in a very little nutmeg and a little fresh parsley, tarragon or basil. Slice over the top 1 or 2 small peeled tomatoes and, if you like, 2 or 3 stoned black olives. Leave to cool.

100. Mushroom Salad

½ lb. mushrooms | *olive oil*
½ a lemon | *seasonings and herbs*

This salad must be made the day before it is eaten. Make a well-mixed dressing of the juice of ½ lemon, 4 tablespoons of olive oil, 1 tablespoon of water, ½ tablespoon of salt, a ¼ teaspoon of sugar, a very little pepper and, if you can get them, finely chopped parsley and tarragon. Wash the mushrooms and put them into the dressing in a container with a top, such as a jar or a plastic storage container. Leave them until the next day, turning the container gently over and about from time to time. Before serving, lift the mushrooms out of any dressing that remains. Curious as the method sounds, it produces tender and well-flavoured mushrooms, of a freshness welcome in a diet where almost nothing is raw.

101. Tomatoes in Cream

A bland and delicious way to serve young tomatoes is to cover them with a dressing simply of cream, slightly salted, and with parsley, chervil or, best of all, tarragon, chopped and mixed into it. If the tomatoes are really tiny, they need only be dipped quickly into boiling water and peeled, but can be left whole. If they are larger it is safer to peel them, halve them, remove the stalk end and with a teaspoon scoop out the seeds from each half. They then look more appealing put flat side down into a dish that just holds them, before the dressing is poured on.

102. Avocado Pears

A really ripe avocado, that must be eaten the day you buy it, is the right kind for the ulcer diet. Such ones are often cheap, too. They need only be halved lengthways, just before eating, have their stones removed, and be served with a dressing of olive oil, lemon juice and salt. A mayonnaise well thinned with lemon juice is a good alternative.

Avocados make convenient picnic food: you take them whole, a knife to open them on the spot, a teaspoon for each person, and the dressing in a bottle.

A friend of delicate stomach does excellently the dish in which you scoop out the pulp of the avocado, gradually beat olive oil into it with a fork, add lemon juice and salt to taste and put the flesh back into the skin. But since the reassembled avocados look sad unless filled to the top, this dish involves starting with more than the usual ½ per person and is therefore expensive.

103. Salad of New Potatoes

1 lb. small new potatoes
olive oil
lemon juice

Potato salad bought from a delicatessen will almost certainly be tinned, have much vinegar in its dressing and therefore be risky. Less easy to explain is the common experience among ulcer sufferers that potato salads in mayonnaise dressings, even home-made ones, sit rather heavily. A further difficulty is that almost all potatoes sold now in England are of the floury kind which fall apart in cooking.

The only potato salad I make is one of small new potatoes, all of a size, boiled in their skins until a skewer will just go through them, skinned, and put hot into a dressing of the juice of ½ lemon with ½ teaspoon of salt dissolved in it, and 3 tablespoons of olive oil. The potatoes should be turned about several times before they are cold and again whenever you are passing. They need at least 2 or 3 hours in the dressing and are better put into it the day before. Finely chopped parsley is an improvement.

Do not, of course, on any account, add raw onion, even the smallest quantity, to a potato salad for an ulcer sufferer.

104. Cauliflower Salad

Remove the cauliflower sprigs from the centre and cut off all hard pieces. Boil in ¼ inch of salted water or, better, steam. When a skewer will go through the stem comfortably (10–12 minutes), drain the pieces, cook, and arrange flowers upward in a dish. Pour over thinned mayonnaise, or boiled salad dressing (p. 141), and scatter chopped parsley on top. This is filling, quite enough, with a hard-boiled egg or two, for lunch on a hot day.

105. A Plate of Young Vegetables

This suggestion is mainly for those who grow their own vegetables, for the moment when these first appear in quantities not big enough to make a whole dish of any one. Only the tiniest will do, but they can be turnips, broad beans, French beans, carrots and should certainly include some very small potatoes. The vegetables should be peeled, scraped or shelled as they require, steamed in separate batches, placed still separate on a large plate and have poured over them a small amount of oil and lemon juice well-mixed together. They should then be served with the cold egg and lemon sauce which follows, and hard-boiled eggs or slices of cold meat.

106. Cold Egg and Lemon Sauce

3 *eggs*
1 *tablespoon oil*
1 *lemon*
1 *teaspoon cornflour*
½ *pint stock*

The stock need be nothing special: the water from steamed or boiled vegetables, or a carrot, an onion, a bay leaf and a couple of peppercorns simmered for ½ hour.

Whisk the eggs in a bowl with the oil, the juice of the lemon and the cornflour dissolved in 2 teaspoons of water. Transfer the mixture to a double saucepan, or bowl fitted into a saucepan, gradually add the warmed stock and stir with a wooden spoon until it thickens a little. Don't expect much thickening, or let the sauce overheat and curdle. Cool and put in the refrigerator for a few hours.

This is good with any cold meat or vegetable; if made for the latter it can employ the cooking water from the vegetable.

107. Boiled Salad Dressing

3 tablespoons flour
1 teaspoon sugar
1 teaspoon salt
1 egg
juice of ½ a lemon
¼ pint water
¼ pint milk
3 tablespoons salad oil

Un-French and quite out of fashion, these pre-war boiled salad dressings have advantages. Lightest and easiest of all to eat for someone with an ulcer, they are quick and simple to make. They are cheap; olive oil is wasted on them and one of the less expensive kinds should be used. They are stable and keep in the refrigerator.

Mix the dry ingredients in the top of a double boiler. Add first the egg, then gradually the lemon juice, milk and water. Cook over boiling water, stirring, until the sauce thickens (only 5–10 minutes), then for another 5. Cool and beat in the salad oil with a wooden spoon.

108. Mayonnaise

2 egg yolks
⅓ pint oil
juice of ½ a lemon
salt

This best of all cold dressings has the reputation of upsetting some stomachs. I, and every possessor of an ulcer I know, find the opposite: that it makes easier the sometimes difficult period of the year when much food is served cold or raw.

Mayonnaise for the ulcer diet should *not*:

1. Be filled with garlic or, in my view, contain garlic at all.
2. Be thinned with vinegar.
3. Be too thick or based upon too much oil added to a single yolk.

Although for ordinary salad dressing olive oil tastes so much the best, any vegetable oil I've used makes a good mayonnaise. I know no dietary argument against peanut or sunflower seed oil, and certainly they are a more sane price than olive oil.

My method of many years standing is to start with 2 yolks absolutely free of white in a dry bowl. I use nothing but a table fork, and a small jug with which to add the oil slowly, stirring in each pouring.

When you have 2 or 3 tablespoons of sauce you can add the oil faster. Have ready the squeezed juice of ½ a lemon with ½ teaspoon of salt dissolved in it. If the sauce gets too thick to work at any time, add a few drops to thin it. Otherwise, at the end, add to the finished mayonnaise enough of the juice to produce a creamy texture. About ⅓ of a pint of oil to 2 yolks produces the right quantity and texture of sauce but you can obviously make more or less.

If the mayonnaise curdles the only course that works for me is to add the curdled mixture slowly to a new yolk in a new bowl. You can keep a mayonnaise for a day in a cool larder; some keep it longer in a refrigerator but mine curdle when I try it.

Many blenders make mayonnaise efficiently and most come with directions for doing it.

Puddings and Sweet Dishes

109. Strawberry fool
110. Gooseberry fool
111. Rhubarb fool
112. Sliced baked apples
113. Stewed apple
114. Poached apples
115. Apple amber
116. Stewed fruit with meringue topping
117. Cherries in syrup
118. Apricot mousse
119. Cold lemon soufflé
120. Orange salad
121. Zwieback pie crust
122. Chocolate mousse
123. Baked bananas
124. Chocolate cake
125. Carrageen
126. Boiled custard

INTRODUCTION

Under this heading only pastry, heavy suet puddings and fritters are warned against for those with ulcers. The skills in cake-making many English women have can be used fully when cooking for someone with an ulcer. Only cakes containing whole nuts, dried or glazed fruits must be avoided. All others are positively encouraged.

If circumstances allow, a piece of cake with tea in the afternoon helps fill the long gap between meals. After main meals stewed fruit, when served with plain cake, is not only nicer but easier on the stomach, I find. The American combination of ice-cream and cake is worth remembering. Some cakes are quite sufficient on their own, such as the one given on p. 155.

Cookery suggestions for puddings for this diet generally include endless variations upon milk, eggs and some thickener such as rice, tapioca or semolina. These milk puddings are, of course, most soothing recourses for troubled periods. Many of them are delicious but too many will pall. There can be no cook who doesn't know how to make them. They are all extremely fattening: therefore harmful, if given in excess, to the ulcer sufferer, and probably unwelcome to others who come to the table with him.

I have therefore not taken up space with them but concentrated upon some less familiar recipes. More of these than is usual in ulcer cookery are based upon the use of fruits in their seasons. These prevent the diet from becoming too stodgy and bring a pleasant sense of order to the table, not to be undervalued for its part in coping with an ulcer.

Many fruits are also potentially dangerous and, like all the most desirable foods for the ulcer diet, require care from the cook—and cash.

All fruits pass from a stage of tart acidity towards the moment of ripeness, when to some degree the acid turns to sugar. If the fruit which the cook uses is not fully ripe, then nothing she can do to it will decrease its acidity. Neither cooking nor sweetening alters the balance of acidity; though both help in less measurable ways to make fruit acceptable to those with ulcers, as anyone who has one knows. So does the presenting of fruit in some bland background such as custard, or cream or a mixture of the two.

In the recipes which follow, I suggest various ways of achieving this. But I repeat that the fruit must be thoroughly ripe to start with. A good measure here is for the cook to use no fruit for preparation in the ulcer diet which she cannot, herself, eat quite happily in its raw state.

Many sources of vitamin C are missing from this diet, or have their content much reduced by cooking. An easy way to balance this is to keep on hand a bottle of rose hip syrup and to use it for the last-minute sweetening which cooked fruit so often demands. Added when the fruit is cool (not before cooking, of course) it makes no difference in taste that I can detect.

Although there is no scientific explanation for this fact, most ulcer sufferers find stewed or other cooked fruit easier on a sensitive stomach when served cold. If plainly stewed or baked, fruit is also safer served accompanied by cream, custard or milk thickened in some such way as the Carrageen recipe which comes in this section. Sponge fingers or other biscuits help, too.

I list here the fruits you are most likely to consider and their place in the ulcer diet.

Apples. No ulcer sufferer should eat raw apples, nor cooking apples, however they are cooked. Ripe eating apples, properly cooked, help to avoid the complete inner standstill to which stodgy food often brings those with ulcers.

Provided you avoid apples sold as cookers altogether, you can use many recipes beyond the few simple ones included here (pp. 149–150): those that combine the apples with bread, in charlottes, or breadcrumbs in such dishes as brown betty, or with egg white in apple snow. Conventional baked apples, with their inedible peel and uneven sweetening, prove unsatisfactory for those with ulcers. When the stomach is troublesome, apple dishes are better served cold, with cream.

Apricots. Really ripe fresh apricots are good baked slowly with vanilla sugar, cooled and served with cream; dried apricots are good for those with ulcers if stewed slowly and made into a purée. See too the recipe on p. 152.

Bananas. Bananas should be on hand at all times in any household where there is an ulcer. They can be eaten at the most difficult times. They are good just as they come but even better sliced, sprinkled with a little sugar in which a piece of vanilla pod is kept and served with cream. See also the recipe on p. 155.

Blackberries. A very few ripe blackberries can be cooked with apples, put through the food mill with them and served cold. In general, a fruit to be avoided and certainly never eaten raw.

Blackcurrants. Blackcurrant drinks are excellent for those with ulcers; otherwise, this fruit should be avoided.

Cherries. Not to be eaten raw but see recipe on p. 151.

Gooseberries. Recommended by some writers on ulcer diet but only at the moment when the fresh ones are really ripe and then cooked as in the recipe I give for them on p. 148.

Grapefruit. To be avoided.

Lychees. A world crop failure occurred during the preparation of this book. Assuming that they reappear, the fresh ones, though troublesome to get out of their husks, are recommended on their own with cream or combined with bananas. Tinned ones are also perfectly safe.

Oranges. See recipe on p. 153.

Peaches. To be avoided.

Pears. When really ripe, one of the few fruits safe eaten raw; they should always be peeled.

Plums. If you can find really ripe, sweet plums they can be stewed for the ulcer diet. The very sour ones generally sold will be upsetting, however treated.

Rhubarb. I find this quite safe as I present it in my recipe (p. 148), and it is recommended by some writers on ulcer cookery. Others are suspicious, so rhubarb should only be served to those who like and report no trouble with it.

Strawberries. Not ideal, but for those who refuse to be deprived, my recipe below is the best way to treat them.

109. Strawberry Fool

1 *lb. strawberries*
¼ *pint double cream*
1 *small carton yoghourt*
1 *egg white*
2 *heaped tablespoons sugar*

Wash the strawberries and remove the stems. Put them through the finest mesh of the Mouli and add the sugar. Beat the cream until it is thick, but not stiff and dry. Add the yoghourt and mix together. Beat egg white until stiff and fold in. Mix in strawberry purée lightly. Chill for 1 hour.

110. Gooseberry Fool

2 lb. ripe fresh gooseberries
¼ pint double cream
*¼ pint thick cooled custard**
8 tablespoons sugar
1 bunch elder flowers

Wash and pick over the gooseberries but don't bother to top and tail them. Put them into a double boiler, or simply into a bowl that will fit into a saucepan.

Add the sugar to the gooseberries *but no water*. Put the head of elder flowers on top, cover and cook until the berries are soft, stirring occasionally (about 45 minutes). Lift out the flower head and discard it. Put the berries through the Mouli.

Chill or simply cool the purée. Just before the meal add to the purée first the custard, blend well. Beat the cream a little—only to thicken it, not until it is stiff. Add this to the mixture and stir well. Taste the fool and add more sugar if necessary. The elder flowers are there to improve the flavour and are optional.

111. Rhubarb Fool

1½ lb. rhubarb
½ pint cream
8 tablespoons sugar

Trim off ends and every scrap of leaf from the rhubarb. Wash and cut it into 1- to 2-inch lengths, preserving all the skin for the sake of its colour. Put rhubarb and sugar, but no water, into a bowl which will fit into a saucepan. Cover the bowl with a lid or plate and cook over boiling water until the rhubarb is soft, which may take ½–1 hour.

When cool put into a blender if you have one; if not, beat

* Made by any method you normally use; or by the one described on p. 156, using ¼ pint milk, 2 egg yolks, 1 tablespoon sugar, and 1 teaspoon cornflour.

with a fork in a bowl until reasonably smooth. Add cream gradually, tasting as you go. Depending on the rhubarb, you may want less than ½ pint, but you certainly won't want more.

Chill until you are ready to serve.

112. Sliced Baked Apples

Not really a recipe, simply a suggestion: when you have the oven on low for some other purpose, use the bottom plate to bake sliced apples which you'll later serve cold. Peel, thoroughly core and slice the apples in rings. Put them into a shallow oven dish with honey, a little water, the juice of an orange. On top put a strip or two of the orange peel, a few seedless raisins, a piece of stick cinnamon. Vary ingredients according to what you have to hand: cloves instead of cinnamon, golden syrup or brown sugar instead of honey. Cover the dish with its lid, or foil, and cook until the apples are just soft, spooning the juice over them once or twice in the cooking.

113. Stewed Apple

This is worth making well, for eating on its own or for use in any recipe that calls for it. I have experimented with dozens of ways, and strongly recommend this one:

2 *lb. apples*	4 *cloves*
4 *tablespoons golden syrup*	*lemon peel*

Wash and core but do not peel the apples. Cut them into quarters and put them into a thick pan with the other ingredients.

Add no water at all: ulcer cookery is quite watery enough without diluting anything unncessarily.

Either cook them in a slow oven for an hour, if you happen

to have it on, or on the lowest possible heat on top for 35–40 minutes. If on top, watch closely and turn over at the beginning so that it does not burn.

Press through the Mouli and let cool.

114. Poached Apples

Delicious and easy, but the timing is critical.

4 *eating apples*
4 *tablespoons golden syrup*
4 *tablespoons water*
1 *dessertspoon butter*
a piece of stick cinnamon

Put the syrup, water, butter and a 1-inch piece of stick cinnamon into a pan with a lid. Cook extremely gently for 15 minutes, taking care not to let it boil dry.

Peel and core the apples, leaving them whole. Put them into the liquid and spoon it over them.

You may cook them either for ½ hour in a slow oven (or on top, on a very gentle heat) for 15 minutes. But in either case too much heat or too long cooking will cause the apples to fall apart. The dish is ready when the apples are soft but before they begin to disintegrate.

If you are going to eat the apples cold, leave out the butter and serve them with cream.

115. Apple Amber

stewed apples
2 *eggs*
2 *tablespoons caster* or *powdered sugar*

Stew about 1½ lb. of apples any way you like but flavour them with something: cinnamon, cloves, lemon peel, vanilla. Let them cool and pour into an ovenproof dish.

Beat the yolks with a fork and then mix well with the stewed apple. Whisk the whites until stiff but not dry, add the sugar, 1 tablespoon at a time, and whisk some more: if you have icing sugar use it instead of caster. Spread quickly over the stewed apple, sprinkle a very little caster sugar on top and bake at 350° for 30 minutes or until top is lightly browned. Good hot, cold or tepid.

116. Stewed Fruit with Meringue Topping

When cookery books say that the preceding recipe can be made with other ingredients, nobody takes this seriously.

But, in fact, the apple amber recipe is an excellent way to serve in the ulcer diet other stewed fruits. Alternatively, a small quantity of dried apricots, soaked, stewed separately and added to the apples, or simply a purée of stewed dried apricots make pleasant variations of the recipe.

117. Cherries in Syrup

1½–2 *lb. cherries*
sugar
1 *tablespoon kirsch, optional*

Don't start with any smaller quantity of cherries: 1½ lb. makes barely enough for 3 or 4 people.

Stone the cherries, which is easy with the gadget made for the purpose, and impossible without. Put 2 tablespoons of sugar for each ½ lb. of cherries into a pan containing a large wineglass of water. Bring this to the boil and put in the cherries. They will take about 3 minutes to come back to the boil and about 7 to cook, gently, until soft.

Lift them out of the juice and reduce it by boiling until it is thick. Pour it over the cherries.

Serve chilled with cream, or hot without it.

If you have redcurrant jelly, substitute 1 tablespoon of it for one of the tablespoons of sugar. If you wish to add kirsch (for a dinner party), put 1 tablespoon into the thickened syrup, leave the heat on for a minute and then leave the syrup to cool before pouring it over the cherries.

118. Apricot Mousse

8 *oz. dried apricots*
¼ *pint cream*
½ *pint milk*
3 *egg yolks*
3 *oz. caster sugar*
½ *oz. gelatine*
juice of ½ *lemon*
almond essence
additional sugar for sauce

Wash the apricots, cover with about twice their volume of water and soak overnight. Cook slowly in the water they soaked in, with a piece of lemon rind. In 20–30 minutes they will be tender. Put them through the Mouli and leave to cool.

Put the gelatine into the lemon juice and 3 tablespoons of water; leave to dissolve.

Heat the milk to boiling point. Mix the egg yolks and sugar smoothly together; add the milk and stir well. Cook, stirring, on a low heat until it just begins to thicken. If the mixture boils it will curdle. When it has cooled add the dissolved gelatine.

Measure ⅜ pint of the apricot purée (keep the rest). Whip the cream only until it begins to thicken, add the measured purée to it and mix lightly. Fold into the custard. Pour into a mould or a bowl the right size, lightly moistened with almond essence.

Boil up 3 tablespoons of sugar and as much water. Add to the remaining apricot purée only as much as will sweeten it adequately and thin it enough to be poured. Put both mousse and sauce into the refrigerator.

Take out the mousse a couple of hours before serving. Only just before, turn it out on to a dish. Take the chilled purée from the refrigerator, pour over the mousse and serve.

119. Cold Lemon Soufflé

3 *large eggs*
½ *lb. caster sugar*
2½ *lemons*
½ *pint cream*
½ *oz. gelatine*

Wash the lemons and pare off with a vegetable peeler a thin layer of their outer skin. Squeeze the juice and put it, the peel, the egg yolks only, and the sugar into a pan. Stir over a low heat for 10–15 minutes until the mixture thickens slightly: never stop stirring or it will curdle. Strain it and whisk as it cools. In about 5 minutes it will be thick and frothy.

Melt the gelatine in 4 tablespoons of water. Lightly whip the cream. Add both to the cooled mixture. Whisk the egg whites and fold them in.

Pour the mixture into a dish it fills to the brim. Or, if you can be bothered, prepare instead a soufflé dish with parchment or greaseproof paper tied around it so that the soufflé will look as though it has risen.

120. Orange Salad

6 *large oranges*
2 *tablespoons granulated sugar*
2 *tablespoons redcurrant jelly*
6 *allspice corns*

Don't use a knife, chopping-board or anything else that is not absolutely clean and free of other food tastes, or these will transfer to the oranges with the disgusting results we have all experienced in restaurants.

Wash 2 oranges well and pare off a thin layer of their peel with a vegetable peeler. Put this, sugar, redcurrant jelly and allspice into 1 pint of water and boil for ½ hour or so with the lid off. Keep the heat low so that it doesn't boil dry.

Meanwhile peel the other oranges and the first two, strip off all the pith you can, slice them thinly, remove pips and arrange in a glass bowl. When the syrup has cooled, strain it and pour it over the orange slices. Keep it in a cool place or refrigerator for a few hours or overnight.

If you lack allspice and redcurrant jelly make the syrup simply with the peel and 4 tablespoons of granulated sugar.

121. Zwieback Pie Crust

Zwieback rusks, about 8
2 dessertspoons sugar
$\frac{1}{2}$ *cup butter*

Pastry made in the conventional way is not recommended for those with ulcers. A better method makes use of the rusks called Zwieback, which good grocers sell.

Cream the butter with a wooden spoon until it is soft. Butter your pie plate and have it nearby. Put the rusks on a board and crush into crumbs with a rolling-pin. Stop when you have 2 cups and mix the sugar with them. Pour this into the bowl with the butter and knead with your fingers until blended. Still with your fingers make the crust in the pie plate, pressing it against bottom and sides.

Bake the crust for 12–15 minutes at 325°.

The idea for this recipe comes directly from *Good Food for Bad Stomachs*, though I have altered it slightly. The crust can be used with any suitable filling: cooked ripe fruits, purées of apricots or prunes, custards flavoured in various ways. The pies can be left open or topped with either meringue or whipped cream.

122. Chocolate Mousse

4 *oz. Menier chocolate*
1 *teaspoon rum, optional*
4 *eggs*

Break up the chocolate and melt it with a tablespoon of water over water that is hot but not boiling. If you happen to have it, add 1 teaspoon of rum. Stir until the chocolate is smooth, let it cool a little and add the 4 beaten egg yolks. Beat the whites until stiff and fold them lightly but thoroughly into the chocolate. When well-mixed pour into a soufflé dish and leave overnight in a cool place.

Popular at a grown-up party this dish is too bitter for most children.

123. Baked Bananas

In cold weather, and on special occasions, this way of baking bananas works well. It will cook in an oven from which a main dish has been removed in the time you take to eat it.

6 *bananas*
1 *large orange*
2 *tablespoons butter*
2 *tablespoons golden syrup*

Place the bananas, peeled and sliced once longways, into a buttered shallow oven dish that just holds them. Pour on the juice of the orange and the golden syrup spread evenly. Cut the butter up over the top. Bake in a moderate oven (350°) for 20 minutes or thereabouts.

124. Chocolate Cake

As readers of this book may well know more about baking than I do, I give only a foolproof recipe for beginners in the field like myself. It is quoted from *French Provincial Cooking* by Elizabeth David, published by Michael Joseph. Since icing a cake is no job for a novice I follow one of Mrs. David's suggestions and serve it with lightly whipped cream instead. Cut small slices, for it is filling.

¼ *lb. bitter chocolate*
¾ *lb. caster sugar*
2 *tablespoons of flour*
3 *eggs*
3 *oz. butter*

'Melt the chocolate in the oven; mix it with the softened butter, flour, sugar and beaten egg yolks. Fold in the stiffly-beaten whites. Turn into a buttered 6-inch cake tin or 1¼-pint loaf tin and cook in a preheated moderate oven, Gas No. 4, 355° F., for 35 minutes. There will be a thin crust on top of the cake but if you test it with a skewer the inside will appear insufficiently cooked, which in fact is correct, as it gets firmer as it cools.

'As soon as it is cool enough to handle, turn upside down on to a cake rack.'

125. Carrageen

⅓ cup carrageen	*¼ teaspoon salt*
3 cups milk	*3 teaspoons sugar*

Whether or not this Irish seaweed confers all the benefits its admirers claim, it thickens satisfactorily and adds a slight but interesting taste to an otherwise unthrilling range of milk puddings. You can buy it at health food stores. This is the basic recipe, for a blancmange good with stewed fruit.

Push the carrageen down hard when measuring the ⅓ cup. Soak in water for 15 minutes and drain. Put into a milk pan with the other ingredients and something to flavour: lemon rind, stick cinnamon, vanilla pod, bay leaf or blade of mace.

Bring slowly to the boil, keep there 3 minutes for a thinnish texture, up to 8 minutes for a stiffer one. Strain and cool.

126. Boiled Custard

3 eggs	*3 tablespoons sugar*
1 teaspoon cornflour	*a piece of vanilla pod* or *vanilla extract*
1 pint milk	

Beat the eggs while the milk comes to the boil. Add the sugar and cornflour to them and whisk a little more. Pour the hot milk over them slowly, stirring with a wooden spoon.

Put into a bowl over just boiling water. Add a piece of vanilla pod (or a little extract) and cook, stirring now and then until the custard coats the spoon. This may take ½ hour or longer. Remove the vanilla pod, if you used one, and chill.

This custard tastes good and improves many puddings but it is only as thick as thin cream and really only good cold.

A thicker one, good either hot or cold, uses exactly the same method, but different proportions:

5 *egg yolks only*
¾ *pint milk*
sugar and vanilla as before

Both are good for the ulcer patient and delicious for anyone: infinitely nicer than the ones made with custard powder. But both, whatever any other cookery book may tell you, are a bore to make: time-consuming and tricky. If the mixture gets too hot it will curdle and is useless.

Appendices

I

BÉCHAMEL OR WHITE SAUCE, AND CHEESE SAUCE

½ pint milk
1½ oz. butter
2 level tablespoons flour
seasonings
for cheese sauce:
2 tablespoons grated cheese

Heat the milk in one saucepan and in another, over a low flame, melt the butter. Add the flour to the butter gradually, and cook for at least 3 minutes. Off the burner, gradually add the heated milk while stirring. Return to the burner, turned low, and stir as it cooks for another 10 minutes. If you have to keep it hot longer, do so by putting the pan into a larger one, in which the water only just simmers.

Notes and variations:

1. If you are going to add no other seasoning, then, when the milk is heating, add to it something to flavour: 4 peppercorns, a bay leaf, a blade of mace, an onion or some fresh herb. Strain these out as you add the hot milk to the sauce.

2. For the milk you may substitute stock or mix these together in various proportions.

3. Taste the sauce near to the time you will serve it and add salt then, not before.

4. If you reheat the sauce do so over hot water.

5. This sauce is used as the basis of many others in this and other cookery books. To make a cheese sauce add to the *cooked* white sauce, as above, 2 tablespoons of finely grated mild English cheese and cook only until the cheese melts.

II

CHEESE

A woman doctor whom I met only once suggested that I should always have in my house a supply of mild English cheese to finish off a meal. It was good advice and I have followed it.

A seldom-mentioned feature of having an ulcer is the feeling that a meal has not been quite adequate: that you are going away from the table still hungry. If nothing is done about the feeling you will almost certainly have a twinge before the next meal. This may be the prelude to real trouble.

Cheese deals well with this difficulty and if it doesn't get eaten quickly it can be used up in cooking. As will appear from many recipes in this book, I favour cheese as a most soothing addition to many dishes.

It must not, obviously, be baked into a hard crust. An old English custom of mixing mustard into cheese cookery is to be avoided, as are a few recipes for incredibly rich dishes combining cheese and cream.

I don't myself suggest for those with ulcers a lunch of bread and cheese alone, finding that this sits heavily.

But with these few reservations cheese has many uses for readers of this book. Both for cooking and eating on its own, I seldom look beyond the English cheeses, which are inexpensive, likely to be in good condition and quite varied: Wensleydale, Caerphilly, Cheshire, Lancashire, Leicester, Derby, Double Gloucester. There is a so-called 'strong' Cheddar which will upset any stomach not made of iron; but many good milder ones which are ideal.

Blue cheeses of any kind may be occasional indulgences but are not for difficult periods; of these, Stilton is less likely to upset than the French or Italian ones.

There are good Dutch and Scandinavian cheeses of the firm kind, and the Italian ones such as Bel Paese are safe.

Although a Frenchwoman of my acquaintance assures me that Camembert is fed to newborn babies, I am cautious of all centre-ripening cheeses. If they are favourites in your house, then the ulcer sufferer should eat only the creamy inside and discard the rind.

All cream cheeses from whatever origin seem to suit ulcers, with the surprising exception of the Boursin with garlic and chives now widely distributed in this country.

Although their flavour adds so much to cookery, both Gruyère and Parmesan have a tendency to clog when melted, so that they must be carefully watched and well-mixed with other ingredients. Small amounts of these cheeses are included in respectable works on ulcer cookery, however, so if you can afford them, use them in this way.

Since fondue sets are selling briskly in this country, I had better say that this lovely sticky concoction is very definitely not for ulcers.

The makers of English cheeses have a highly-organized publicity organization, The Cheese Bureau, 40 Berkeley Square, London, W.1. They publish recipe collections which contain some inexpensive dishes suitable for the ulcer diet, either as they stand or with slight modifications.

Here is a summary to help with the choosing of English cheeses:

Caerphilly. Mild, and to be recommended.

Cheddar. To be chosen with extreme care, and never ordered by this name alone: Canadian and other very strong Cheddars can be upsetting.

Cheshire. Both red and white forms safe, and recommended; the blue form is good for an occasional indulgence.

Derby. Best eaten when young, as the mature cheese develops too strong a character.

Double Gloucester. A little care in choosing is necessary, as there are some over-strong forms of it to be bought.

Lancashire. This cheese is available in mild, medium and strong forms, and only the mild one is to be recommended.

Leicester. A safe choice, and a good one.

Stilton. In its blue form, the best of the veined cheeses for those with ulcers; and in its rarer white form, a safe and interesting cheese.

Wensleydale. With Caerphilly, the safest buy as neither has, as far as I know, any but mild-flavoured forms.

Processed Cheeses. Blended cheese is always an innocuous choice. I would, therefore, when in a situation where doubtful of other cheeses, rely on one of these.

III

WHAT TO DRINK

At breakfast, and indeed at any time, drink tea rather than coffee; drink it not too strong and with milk. Make full use of the wide variety of teas available in this country.

Chocolate and other drinks dissolved in hot milk should be on hand for the between-meals and bedtime drinks every ulcer sufferer should have. Cold milk and flavoured milk drinks should certainly be encouraged for those who like them. If you have a blender you can use it to produce a pleasant range of these, by mixing milk with fruit syrups, bananas and other things suggested in the instructions that come with most blenders.

Ulcer sufferers are short of good drinks to accompany meals. Blackcurrant drinks, Ribena and some of its less expensive competitors, were found in one group of experiments to be particularly suitable. I have found them both pleasant and safe.

Other concentrated fruit squashes are less reliable, as many have a high acid content. There is an excellent, but expensive, range of German, non-alcoholic fruit drinks beginning to be available here.

Alcoholic Drinks

The most positive advice I have to give is this: ask your doctor, directly and plainly, for his orders and follow them.

Having said this, in an area of some controversy, I can only summarize those I have received from my own doctor.

1. *Do not drink spirits at all.* This means what it says, quite simply.

2. Drink very little of anything alcoholic, wine, beer or whatever, and drink it only at mealtimes.

3. At mealtimes means when the food is on the table, not for two hours beforehand. Avoid at all costs a prolonged pre-meal drinking session.

If you attend cocktail parties and refuse the drink offered, your host may well offer you some non-alcoholic alternative, which he is not to know will be almost as bad for you as the alcohol; tonic water, bottled fruit or tomato juices, bitter lemon, all are acid and potentially upsetting. Plain water, with ice and a small slice of lemon, makes a drink that looks convincing. But on such a drink cocktail parties aren't much fun, and ulcer sufferers avoid them, if they can.

Effervescent drinks are suspect and therefore a still, draught beer is a better choice than a bubbly one from a bottle, and brown ales and stouts than lighter beers.

I had intended to include in this book a table of wines of low acid content to be recommended to those with ulcers. I asked for the help of Mr. Colin Fenton of the wine department of Sotheby's, and he in turn told me that research into the acid content of wines was at that moment being conducted by Mr. R. W. Goswell, Chief Chemist of John Harvey & Sons Ltd.

Mr. Goswell has most generously summarized his work for my use. Its general purport is that such a table as I pictured would be impractical, and even perhaps dangerous, since it might lead some readers to think that there were truly safe wines. Although perfectly safe for normal stomachs, all wines contain, in Mr. Goswell's words, 'more acid than would be desirable for sufferers from this complaint'. The differences are minimal and vary in wines from the same district from year to year.

Mr. Goswell does, however, confirm an observation common among ulcer sufferers, and which has been reported to me by a consultant at a London teaching hospital: that red wines from the more southerly regions of Europe—red Burgundies, red Rhone wines, Italian reds, Spanish reds—

are marginally safer. But these margins are small. Expert advice, and my own, is to treat wine-drinking as an occasional pleasure, not a regular habit. Large firms and groups such as the Wine Society, will give advice on choice from their current stocks.

A final warning. Eschew the champagne offered at christenings, or at weddings; even your own, unless you want to spend an ulcerated honeymoon.

IV

BREAKFAST

The worst possible way for someone with an ulcer to begin the day is, I suspect, one of the most common: a cup of black coffee and nothing else.

It matters less, within reason, what you eat in the morning than that you eat something. In a busy house with children leaving for school and offices to be reached on time it is not easy to organize the substantial and varied breakfast menus that undoubtedly do the most good. I limit myself to these few, I hope, realistic suggestions.

1. Tea is a better breakfast drink than coffee. It should be freshly made, not too strong and fairly milky. If you insist on drinking coffee, which you definitely should not, drink little of it and put in plenty of milk. A milk-based drink, such as hot chocolate, is best of all for those who will consider this unconventional idea.

2. Never drop below this basic minimum: a boiled egg and 2 pieces of toast. Poached eggs take scarcely longer. Eggs scrambled in a double saucepan make a pleasant change.

3. If you like cereals, include them, hot or cold. Hospital kitchens sieve porridge for those on gastric diets, but for the purposes of this book the oats treated to make them cook quickly are perfectly acceptable. Among dry packaged cereals avoid the very fibrous ones such as All-Bran.

4. Time-setting ovens can be useful in providing occasional changes to breakfast menus. Pre-set at 350° (or whatever the instructions with your cooker say), they cook bacon most successfully, and by the method most widely recommended in works on ulcer diet. The same method works well for smoked haddock cooked in milk.

5. Fresh fish plainly baked in milk is another good break-

fast dish for someone with an ulcer. So is kedgeree, but I don't see this being served regularly in any house I know!

6. I personally find fruit juices too sharp for me at breakfast, but they are sanctioned by every writer on diet I have read, so they can certainly be included if you like them. To make them slightly softer to the taste, bring, only just, to the boil or dilute with boiling water, then cool.

7. Marmalade which contains large pieces of peel should be avoided. Other marmalades, jams, and particularly honey, are better.

Above all, get up in time to sit down and eat something reasonable. To gulp and run, every day, will undo much of what a sensible diet can otherwise do for someone with an ulcer.

V

EATING BETWEEN MEALS

'Little and often' is the catch-phrase widely associated with the correct eating pattern for those with ulcers. I suggest that readers of this book treat it with some scepticism; or rather, think carefully about what it involves.

No ulcer sufferer should ever miss a meal. No ulcer sufferer should ever eat gargantuan meals. But equal dangers lurk in nibbling biscuits and sipping milk for the whole of every day.

Ulcers in the phase requiring hospital treatment certainly were, and doubtless in some places are, fed on nothing but small quantities of milk for long periods. This book is not for such people.

If you have had an upsetting incident of some kind, or a missed meal, or been given something unsuitable to eat, then you may well take to bed for a day, when you will eat little, and drink milk or milk drinks. But for a day only: an ulcer sufferer can have milk and biscuits thrust at him too often.

They do not constitute a well-balanced diet for an extended period. They will lead to constipation, to lethargy and loss of interest in other food. What is almost worse, they will put the ulcer sufferer out of phase with the rest of his family in matters of food.

The aim of every ulcer sufferer, and of his wife, should be to fit in with normal mealtimes. Ordinary meals with others can, and should be, supplemented by something in between them: in the morning, a glass of milk, or a cup of milky tea and a biscuit, and in the afternoon, tea and a piece of cake. At bedtime, milky tea or a milk drink is useful.

Those who work in offices should be firm about demanding the right to a morning and afternoon break for these purposes. The desk, or the suitcase on a journey, should always contain a box of biscuits in case of emergency.

But nobody can live on biscuits. Even milk has its limitations for an adult. If they take away the appetite for all other food they are false friends to someone with an ulcer.

VI

MEASUREMENTS AND OVEN TEMPERATURES

In this book 1 cup means the standard English measuring cup holding 10 fluid oz., and 1 pint the standard English one of 20 oz.

Most measurements under ½ lb. in this book are given in tablespoons because even the best kitchen scales are inexact for these small quantities. But for those who prefer to weigh, here are some rough approximations:

1 oz. butter or fat = 2 tablespoons
1 oz. caster sugar = 2 tablespoons
1 oz. sifted flour = 4 tablespoons

I give below a chart of equivalent readings for gas and electric ovens. Those who, like me, use the latter, will probably find an oven thermometer a much better guide to temperatures than the figures on the controls.

Electricity	*Gas*
240°–310°	¼–2
320°–370°	3–4
380°–400°	5
410°–440°	6–7
450°–500°	8–9

Bibliography

with notes on useful books for further reading

I. General Advice to those with Duodenal Ulcers

How to Live with your Duodenal Ulcer. Robert Kemp, M.D., M.R.C.P. The British Medical Association, 1956.

Making Friends with your Ulcer. Robert Kemp, M.D., M.R.C.P. *A Family Doctor Booklet.* The British Medical Association, 1960.

The first title is a book, the second a pamphlet explaining the sensible approach to a duodenal ulcer. This advice seems to me essential reading. The booklet can be obtained from the British Medical Association, Tavistock Square, London, W.C.1.

II. Ulcer Diet and Convalescent Cookery

Practical Diet for Peptic Ulcers. Richard Barrymore, M.D. Arthur Barker Ltd., 1964.

Good Food for Bad Stomachs. Sara M. Jordan, M.D. and Sheila Hibben. With an introduction by Harold W. Ross. Doubleday & Co. Inc., 1951.
In my knowledge the first book devoted wholly to cooking for an ulcer. Harold Ross, editor of the *New Yorker* magazine, suggested this collaboration between one of his cookery con-

tributors and the doctor who treated his ulcer. Even though American in point of view, and more restricted than most current thinking on ulcer diet in this country, a book well worth owning if you have a way to get it. Still in print in the U.S.A.

Invalid Cookery Book. Marguerite Patten. Phoenix House, 1953.
Recommended by Dr. Kemp. Principally about the practicalities of preparing and serving food to invalids, this contains one section of 'Dishes for Gastric Patients'.

Cooking for Special Diets. Bee Nilson. Penguin Books, 1964.
An authoritative work by the distinguished dietician and cookery writer, this treats the ulcer diet among a number of others.

Nutrition and Diet Therapy. Agnes E. Pavey, S.R.N. Faber and Faber Ltd., 1948.

The Ulcer Diet Cook Book. Harold Rubin. With an introduction by Franz J. Lust, M.D., L.F.A.C.G. George Allen and Unwin Ltd., 1968.
This American volume, also by an ulcer sufferer, appeared when my own was half finished. The range of foods permitted is narrower than that generally allowed in this country. The book appears to have been printed unrevised from American plates and so contains references to bluefish, butterfish and other foods either unknown or unavailable in Great Britain. Nonetheless, a pleasant book which would be useful in the early stages of recovery from an attack.

Recipes for Light Diets. E. M. Shipley and H. M. Dundas. J. & A. Churchill Ltd., 1951.
Recommended by Dr. Kemp. A pamphlet containing about forty pages of very simple, sensible recipes.

Handbook of Diets. Rose M. Simmonds, S.R.N. William Heinemann (Medical Books) Ltd., 1937.

III. General Cookery Books

First Slice Your Cookbook. Arabella Boxer. Nelson, 1964.
Many people with ulcers find this book, with its high proportion of simple and lightly seasoned dishes, the most useful one to have appeared recently. Its companion, *A Second Slice*, contains few recipes suitable for the ulcer diet.

Good Fish from the Sea. Helen Burke. André Deutsch, 1965. With a foreword by the Chairman of the White Fish Authority.
Recommended to me by the White Fish Authority, the best up-to-date treatment of fish cookery I discovered, with many useful recipes and much good advice.

Deep Freezing. Pat M. Cox. Faber and Faber. 1968.
Although I have not frozen food myself, I believe this book to be the best on the subject.

Summer Cooking. Elizabeth David. Museum Press, 1955.
Of all Mrs. David's books this has the best selection of recipes usable by those with ulcers. But no one who cooks in this country should be without any of her works. *French Provincial Cooking* contains many good, simple recipes for soups, egg and cheese dishes, vegetables and ways of treating lamb, veal and poultry. *Italian Food* has an indispensable section on pasta. The first volume in her new series on English Cooking, Ancient and Modern, although concerned with *Spices, Salt and Aromatics in the English Kitchen*, contains some interesting recipes safe for those with ulcers.

Rice Cooking. Robin Howe. André Deutsch, 1959.
This contains a full explanation of the various kinds of rice and of the many viable approaches to cooking it. I have not tried any of the recipes.

The Penguin Cookery Book. Bee Nilson. Penguin Books, 1952.
In my view the best general cookery book ever published in this country, this volume has gone in and out of print over the years since it was published. It contains many recipes for simple dishes which other cookery books do not think worth setting down but which are important to those catering for an ulcer. A new edition, revised by Mrs. Nilson, has been published recently.

Guide to Good Food and Wine, compiled by André L. Simon. Collins, 1952.
This volume which sounds so off-puttingly devoted to high living is in fact an alphabetical reference book divided into sections on sauces, vegetables, cereals, fruit, fish, meat, birds and eggs, cheese and wine, which were originally printed as separate volumes. These vary enormously in quality, even in accuracy, but the ones on fish and on cereals contain information not easy to come by elsewhere.

The Constance Spry Cookery Book. Constance Spry and Rosemary Hume. J. M. Dent & Sons Ltd., 1967.
Contains some traditional English recipes not otherwise easy to find, for good simple food.

Index

Index

Index

Index